AWAKENING TO DISABILITY

Nothing about Us without Us

Karen G. Stone

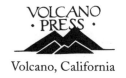

VOLCANO
· PRESS ·

Volcano, California

Karen G. Stone or Volcano Press does not assume liability for damage, injury, or expense incurred as a result of the use of this publication.

Published 1997 by Volcano Press, Inc.
Copyright © 1997 by Karen G. Stone

Library of Congress Cataloging-in-Publication Data
Stone, Karen G., 1946–
    Awakening to disability : nothing about us without us / by Karen G. Stone.
      p.   cm.
    ISBN 1-884244-14-9 (pbk.)
    1. Physically handicapped—United States. 2. Physically handicapped—United States—Life skills guides. I. Title.
HV3023.A3S76   1997
362.4—dc21   97-2096
                                           CIP

Alternative Cataloging-in-Publication Data
Stone, Karen G., 1946–
    Awakening to disability: nothing about us without us. Volcano, CA: Volcano Press, copyright 1997.
    "From . . . columns . . . in the Albuquerque Journal and . . . Miami Herald."
    PARTIAL CONTENTS: A few facts. On disability and language. Invisible disabilities. Visible disabilities. –Some practical matters. Children and disabilities. Women and disabilities. Significant others and friends. Education. Accessible housing. Transportation. Recreation and leisure. Attendant care. Again. Diet, exercise, and health. On the job. Sex. Suicide. –On becoming savvy and then some. Mentors, mentorship, and other admirals. Money and change. –Life after a wheelchair.
    PARTIAL APPENDICES: How to make a public event accessible. –How to effectively deal with injustice.

    1. Disabilities. 2. Disabled persons. 3. Disabled persons—Self-help materials. 4. Disabled persons—Interpersonal relations. 5. Disabled persons—Sexuality. 6. Disability culture. 7. Women wheelchair users—Personal narratives. 8. Disabled workers. 9. Disabled persons—Health. 10. Disabled persons—Recreation. 11. Nonhandicapist language. 12. Disabled persons—Rights. I. Title. II. Title: Nothing about us without us. III. Volcano Press.
362.4

Cover design by Tom Jackson
Text design by David Charlsen
Front cover art: Beloved Aire © 1996, by Sara Steele, All Rights Reserved
Composition by Jeff Brandenburg/ImageComp

To order additional copies of AWAKENING TO DISABILITY, please send $14.95. For postage and handling, add $4.50 for the first book and $1.50 for each additional book. California residents please add appropriate sales tax. Contact Volcano Press for quantity discount rates, and for a current catlaog.

Volcano Presss, Inc. PO Box 270, Volcano, CA 95689
Web address: http://www.volcanopress.com
E-mail: sales@volcanopress.com
For orders: (800) 879-9636   Fax (209) 296-4995
Printed in the U.S.A.

To my family
Who has done so much to keep me alive . . .
Thank you Mom, Dan, and Adam

And to Dad
Whose heart resonates throughout . . .

Acknowledgements to: All ADAPT members of my region, Dr. Patch Adams, Paul Allen, Muthu Barry, Richard Benison, Steve Brock, Ph.D., Lillian Gonzales Brown and Steve E. Brown, Dorie Bunting, Betty Carson, Lois Castillo, Dr. Harold Cohen, Linda Crabtree, Justin Dart, Jeff Dodd, Karuna Fluhart, Carla Garcia, Eda Gordon, David Grady, Ellen Harland, Tom Harmon, Judy Heumann, Kevin Irvine, Kathy Jackson and all my ex-coworkers at Holmes & Narver, Inc., Norma Kwestel, Barbara LaValley, Stephen and Ondrea Levine, the late Kirk MacGugan, Carol Merrill, Skip Miller and Liz Cunningham, Pat Murphy, Ph.D., Kathy Olson, Margaret O'Neal, Dr. Oswaldo Pereira, Leau Phillips, my Quaker family, Tania Ramalho, Adolf and Doro Ratzka, Sara V. Rhodes, Pat Simmons, Cirrelda Snider and J.B. Bryan, Jean Stewart, Dr. Steve Tolber and Louise Campbell, Charlotte Toulouse, Avis and Dyck Vermilye, Wendy Watson, and to the entire Volcano Press staff, David Charlsen, and Zoe Brown.

Last, but not at all least, hats off to Herb Caen who gave me the writer's eye; to Natalie Goldberg who took the eye, turned it into a voice and helped me sing; to Libby Atkins and Martha Trollin who gave me the space to sing my song freely; and to Bob Alberti who encouraged me to believe in my writing a very long time ago.

CONTENTS

Foreword ix

Introduction xi

Part One: A Few Facts
1 On Disability and Language 3
2 Seeing the Barriers 9
3 Invisible Disabilities 27
4 Invisible-to-Visible Disabilities. 51
5 Visible Disabilities 67
6 Chronic Illnesses and Disabilities 75

Part Two: Some Practical Matters
7 Children and Disabilities 83
8 Women and Disabilities 91
9 Significant Others and Friends 99
10 Education 105
11 Accessible Housing 115
12 Transportation. 129
13 Recreation and Leisure 133
14 On Travel, Vacations, Naps, and Then Some . . . 147
15 Attendant Care 157
16 Aging 167
17 Diet, Exercise, and Health 171
18 On the Job. 179
19 Sex. 187
20 Suicide. 193

Part Three: On Becoming Savvy and Then Some

21 Mentors, Mentorship, and Other Admirals . . . 199
22 Parking, Wars, and Other Battles 209
23 Money and Change 215
24 The Last Stop 221
25 A Few Words on Becoming Savvy 229

Part Four: Life after a Wheelchair

26 The Rise after the Stumble 237
27 On Exercising Your Spiritual Muscle 245

Appendices

A How to Make a Public Event Accessible 253
B How to Effectively Deal with Injustice 259
C Discussion Topics for Sex and Disabilities . . . 265

Notes 269

As has often been said, we should not seek limitation, but liberation. We should not reject anything before we have made exerted efforts to find something else. It is better to regard death as being worse than life than to regard life as being worse than death. Even if only once. And only in a free place can anything grow again. What is free seeks enrichment in everything and lets life influence it through all presences—even if it is only a spent match. Only in freedom can what is coming be received.

—Wassily Kandinsky

We have had the privilege of knowing Karen Stone for a little over two years. During that time, we have read many of her newspaper columns, have spent a little time at her wonderfully accessible house, and have followed some of her triumphs and travails.

In *Awakening to Disability: Nothing about Us without Us*, everyone has the chance to spend a little time with Karen. Reading her prose is akin to sitting in her living room and having a conversation. Her voice comes through her essays as clearly as it vibrates in her own home.

This is good news because Karen is writing about topics that are important to everyone. Some of her subjects will seem warm and familiar or cold and daunting to those of us with disabilities who have shared similar experiences. Other topics will be breathtaking and adventurous to all of us, whether or not we share the personal experience of disability.

While reading *Awakening to Disability*, we often felt we were on a journey. This book does what we all need to be doing: it talks about the experience of disability in our lives. This experience adds so much flavor—some pleasant and some not—to our lives, yet most of us rarely speak of it at length. This book chronicles the journey from disability shame to disability pride, not only for the author, but for us all. Our experiences may not be the same, but our feelings are universal.

The gift of this book is not only the thoughts it provokes in the reader, but the door it opens to encourage a dialogue between the disabled and nondisabled. Here the experience of disability can be explored in both the positive and difficult aspects without resorting to histrionics. This kind of dialogue is essential if those of us with disabilities are ever to live with equality in society. We are not the "problem," and we are not "weak." If you have any doubt about that, read on.

Karen does a wonderful job of describing experiences that are extraordinary for some and ordinary for others, while putting a human face on them. The most positive accolade we can give this book is that it held our interest from beginning to end. After reading numerous books and articles on the subject of disability, maintaining our interest from beginning to end rarely happens now.

We invite readers to share this book with those around them. Use it as a guide for discussion groups, as a perspective on disability for parents of children who have disabilities, for disabled youths, for newly disabled folks — or for your own growth. Part of the richness of our disability culture is that we can celebrate a lifestyle that is perceived by so many as a tragedy. There is so much reason for our pride — so much strength in our community. Read on and see if you don't agree.

If that happens, then there will be a chance that, one day, there will be "nothing about us without us." We hope you enjoy this book as much as we did.

Lillian Gonzales Brown
Steven E. Brown
Founders, *Institute on Disability Culture*

INTRODUCTION

After seven plus years of writing about disability issues on a regular basis for a newspaper, I thought writing a book educating, advocating, and inspiring the readers would be a breeze. Nope. I am wrong. Very.

Imagine what it is like taking off in a spaceship. At lift-off, you first might see the launch pad area, then the nearby city, then the state and how that is located within the United States, then how our continent fits in with the other continents and the oceans. Finally, you are looking at the entire globe, the galaxy surrounding it, and the infinite universe beyond. How do you describe that in a few chapters?

Describing the disability experience is like trying to describe the universe from out there or like an Afro-American person trying to convey the black experience to any white person. It is rather challenging, mildly put. And to do it in a relatively few words is daunting, because, in reality, we are describing lifetimes, some old, and some new.

As it happened, just as I began this writing project, my health made a steep dive, and I entered the maelstrom of long-term care challenges. This experience in itself warrants a book. I went from a series of emergency room visits, to a short nursing home stay, to hiring live-in care—all with the financial help of my family, and with the spirited rescue of dear friends.

With a friend's laptop computer, I was able to carry on—the mind clear, the body sagging. Being at the receiving end of care has allowed me to witness and experience first-hand the frailties of our health care system. It has been an incredibly stressful period in my life. And amazingly, despite all, I have gotten well. I attribute a great deal of this to my family's help, the tremendous outpouring of love and support from surrounding friends, and my live-in help.

However, this whole experience has been akin to a large boulder rolling into a small creek. My path, or direction of flow if you will, irrevocably has seen a change.

Nursing home nightmares, especially those experienced by persons with disabilities, are true realities, not stories made up to titillate the public. Abusive treatment does occur. For those at home with hired care, abandonment—leaving the person with a disability, alone and helpless—does happen to many, yours truly included. And, of course, business people see this situation as a most opportune moment to prey, and with relish, they do.

In the duration of two short months, I have changed, changed mightily. What have been heresy, headlines, and exposés on television shows such as "PrimeTime Live," "48 Hours," and "20/20" have become the personal reality. And the personal has become the political. Actually, separating the reality from the stories is like seeing a desert without cactus: a bit strange.

Protesting one of the nation's larger nursing home businesses located a five-minute drive from my home and office, a business that is currently under investigation by the FBI for fraud, I had my wrists slapped by one of the newspapers I write for.

"You are either a columnist or an activist," one of the senior editors told me. Realizing, with this ultimatum, that I can reach more through my written words than my activities, I bit the bullet and said that my choice would be to continue to scribe.

But, what a loaded gun. Memories of lousy hired health-care workers, abusive treatment, nursing home nightmares, greedy business people, abandonment, unaware case workers, and more, have left a bitter taste in my mouth.

Ironically, during this episode, the National Easter Seal Society honored one of my columns, in which I touched on some of these very issues six months prior to experiencing them firsthand. It is the second time I've received such an honor from them. Called the EDI Award, it stands for Equality, Dignity, and Independence. A good one. I stand—oops, sit—for the same qualities. That is what this book is about.

Persons with disabilities call the able-bodied, "TABs."That stands for Temporarily Able-Bodied. Don't laugh. It could not be more valid. I fell into that category royally. Once very physically active and working full time, I now utilize a wheelchair due to multiple sclerosis. The change occurred rapidly. Because of the unpredictability of this chronic illness, a Ph.D. in Copability was required in an equally rapid period. And I learned that finding the ability to cope does not end with any sense of completion. It is an ongoing process, a process many of us share and/or are currently experiencing.

With an interest in architecture, with hands-on experience in home building, with photography and writing skills, and now with a disability, I received two travel grants to photograph and document accessible, but *aesthetic,* home design. This involved travel to Canada and the Scandinavian countries, where design practice has put these countries into the forefront of such architectural progress.

Now, like writer Andre Dubus who writes of his experiences after losing a leg due to an accident, I use words to cross over barriers. When first writing back in 1988, I said: "It is not that we, as persons with disabilities, want to be like the able-bodied any more. Simply, we cannot revert to our former selves or change our bodies. We want, instead, to create a new consciousness and thinking for society . . . and invite the able-bodied to share it with us."

While in Scandinavia, I learned of their five categories of disabilities: mobility impairment, blindness, deafness, mental illness, and allergies. Sadly, in America, we do not consider allergies disabling. If we were to consider all the categories of disabilities utilized by the Scandinavian countries, the figure currently claimed by the latest United States census of 50 million Americans with disabilities — or twenty percent of the population — is an understated estimate. Very underestimated, if you ask me.

The figure, 50 million disabled Americans, largely includes those with obvious disabilities. It is hard to count those with invisible disabilities. Take a person with environmental sensitivity, for example. Are these individuals, disabled by the man-made environment, included in the count? Just addressing persons with obvious disabilities is merely dealing with the tip of the iceberg. We are all touched, somehow, in some way, at some time.

Initially, I was troubled by the difficulty of getting current and conclusive data in the research for this book. I felt frustrated about the lack of timeliness in my presentation of facts. Then I read a scholarly journal covering disability issues, and their data primarily came from the same time frame, if not the same source. This made me realize that current and conclusive data regarding disability issues, though sorely needed, is not considered a high priority. Fortunately, this is changing.

Interestingly, the older reports I garner information from, especially for Chapter 11 on accessible housing, reveal a historical timeliness. You become aware of just how far back in time other countries have grappled with issues involving their disability communities. The Scandinavian countries, in particular, are legendary for their sensitivity to disability issues.

Time and time again, members of the disability community tell me horror stories of how they have been treated in hospitals, rehabilitation centers, and nursing homes. Having personally experienced a few such incidents myself, I know there is no exaggerating here. As Linda Crabtree, founder of *It's Okay!* magazine (see Chapter 19) states, ". . . as far as they are concerned, it [the way the working profession assumes they know better and treats us] is everything about us, without us!"

Having been on both sides of the river, and crossing over by wading in the water at times, swimming or riding the rapids with the help of a life preserver at other moments, I can now knowingly write about the experiences of becoming, and being, disabled. My experience has shaped how I came up with the four parts found in this book. The first part is factual, educational material that will be most useful for the concerned able-bodied community. The second part, the major section of the book, addresses issues that many persons with disabilities face. The third part deals with my own, and ultimately, your own awakening as to what disablement can, or does, mean. And lastly, part four reveals the hard-earned happiness and contentment reaped after all these years. Yes, there is life after a wheelchair.

Awakening to Disability: Nothing about Us without Us is about the *human* aspects of the disability experience; it is not a legal treatise on the ways and means of disability know-how. There are plenty of such books and articles already written.

I personally wish I could have had such a book to read when experiencing the first signs of disability, to know there was life after a wheelchair—to share with others, so they would understand a few of the challenges I was facing at the time. Then I could have given such a book to others, saying, "Here, read this. You'll better comprehend what I am dealing with right now."

People ask how my life after disability (A.D.) changed me. To that, I say it has and it has not. Most important is the person that I am, I still am, and will always be, regardless. What has changed is how I do things, the planning, the process, the consequences. Also, I have become more aware, more political, and certainly closer to my spiritual self and purpose in life. Too, my career has changed. I've gone from a professional photographer, a marketing person, to a full-time writer.

Undoubtedly, as with a mid-life crisis, the changes were challenging and, at times, difficult, painful, and daunting.

I would not wish this upon anyone. But ironically, for all that has happened, I would not change a thing. Granted, I'm slower and have joined the turtle kingdom in that respect. But being disabled has not changed the essential me. The joy of simply being has always been part of my makeup, part of my life.

Many, many people ask me where I find my "joie de vivre." Quite frankly, the question always stumps me. And it still does. True, I now use wheels instead of shoes. But you want to know something? I also still enjoy good key lime pie, the 49ers, and a great joke.

PART ONE

A Few Facts

1

ON DISABILITY
AND LANGUAGE
Welcome to the Club

Whether you are a person with a disability, newly acquired or from birth, or an able-bodied person, there are some common qualities we all share.

Perhaps the most important is that we are all human. Being a member of that club, we all share similar attributes, regardless of background, upbringing, age, ability, sex, or nationality. One shared attribute in particular is a tendency to become less able to do something physically or mentally, due to illness, accident, genetics, or age. So? ? ?

Some of us have dark hair, some of us have fair skin, some of us are chubbier than others, some of us come from poor families or no family at all. So? ? ? Regardless, we *all* laugh, cry, have bad days, enjoy a good meal.

Because of societal standards, many nondisabled persons around the globe, appropriately labeled TABs (remember, that stands for the "Temporarily Able-Bodied"), view individuals with disabilities—or those individuals newly disabled—with pity or as part of a horror story. Many people who are, or are becoming, disabled simply are considered less than okay or "less than . . ."

3

Who establishes these guidelines? Who defines an "okay" status? And with all the variety among members of our humankind club, can a normal parameter even encompass all the variations? I ask, is your mother, father, companion, child, or friend really less human because he or she may be considered "less than normal, less than okay?" And tell me, what is even regarded "normal?"

Victor Papanek, Austrian-born author, designer, and world-leading ideologist, asks, "How much of our lives are without some disability?" Take the ordinary. A pregnant woman is slower, and so too is a small child. A student breaks a leg and temporarily ends up in a wheelchair and/or uses crutches for a while. An elderly parent needs to move in with you or vice versa. Papenek estimates that "A person has about ten years when, not involved in a car accident or struck by disease, physical or spiritual, s/he is completely unencumbered." Papanek further states, "Eighty percent of the population are old, obese, small, tall, disabled, in the eight or ninth month of pregnancy, in other words, beyond the 'normal man.'"

Or do I need to remind you of another set of statistics released in December, 1995, at the United Nations on the International Day of Disabled Persons? What was revealed is that one in four families worldwide has a disabled member and one in five people worldwide is disabled, most of them impoverished.

Currently, approximately 50 million Americans, or twenty percent of the population, are considered "less than normal." The numbers, however, are not completely revealing. As previously mentioned, there is more. Much more.

There are the related and affected wives, husbands, lovers, parents, and children of people who have a disability. That is not counting the caregivers, healers, and/or professionals who also might be involved. Add the elderly. It goes without saying, as our younger population grays, so do our parents.

These parents are, because of age, in greater need of assistance in one form or another. Too, are not "those folks" ultimately "us folks?" Or do I need to remind you that, outside of the ever so predictable taxes and death, we all are getting older?

And with age comes the lousy, but unavoidable, marriage with decreasing ability. Welcome to the club, regardless. You are a bona fide member whether you choose to be or not.

Because this club has proven to be so universal in its wide-ranging inclusion, any discussion about disability issues here applies to all of us, eventually. The line drawn between persons with, and persons without, disabilities is far finer than it appears. Our needs are more interchangeable than realized. In fact, a European edition of the *Wall Street Journal* had a front page article covering, as their headline says, "Design for the Elderly Appeals to the Young, Too." I am not surprised.

On Language

While addressing the universality of the disability experience, I'd like to say a bit about the use of damaging language when talking about the disability experience. Numerous people ask me about the correct language when referring to a person with a disability. With the 1990 passage of the Americans with Disability Act here in America, awareness of disability issues remains high. The debate over language, or labeling people to be more precise, is intense; but there is a much-lauded desire among many individuals to be "politically correct."

In fact, there was a contest involving the issue of "Cripplespeak," so to speak. The $50,000 winner came up with "people with differing abilities," a phrase, ironically, not considered very acceptable by the disability community. Why not? Generally, the consensus among the disability community simply is to emphasize the person. Say, "a *person* with a disability," "a *person* who has muscular dystrophy," "a *person* who uses a wheelchair,"— or for example, "an American with a disability." After all, when was the last time you said, "a glassed person" when referring to someone who wears glasses?

Why even identify a person by a disability? Sure, I may not have very functional legs, but I also do not have blond hair. So why make a big issue about my not-so-blond hair? I have never been called "not-so-blond Karen."

Take the word "handicap." To use this word for horse races may be okay, but basically, it is passé in describing a person. Its origin is cap-in-hand, or, to be more explicit, it means begging with a cap in one's hand. Applying such a term to a working person who may be blind is not really appropriate. Simply, a working person does not beg. A working person who has low vision is not considered a beggar either.

Why is the H-word ("handicap") still being used? Back in 1993, the United Nations spelled out fundamental concepts on disability policy, and in doing so, came the closest to a good definition of the H-word. In this publication, the UN says,

> The term "handicap" means the loss or limitation of opportunities to take part in the life of the community on an equal level with others. It describes the encounter between the person with a disability and the environment. The purpose of this term is to emphasize the focus on the shortcomings in the environment and in many organized activities in society. . .

And the UN goes on to say,

> The term "disability" summarizes a great number of different functional limitations occurring in any population in any country of the world. People may be disabled by physical, intellectual or sensory impairment, medical conditions or mental illness.[1]

As a result, every organization I know of—and there are a few across the nation—has dropped the H-word from their name. You know the trend: people first, not labels first.

Meanwhile, "handi-capable" was trounced in *The Disability Rag*,[2] a hard-nosed, clearheaded publication we should all read. *The Rag*, in covering current disability issues, did a survey to learn what their readers thought about various words used to describe people with a disability. One reader said, "'handi-capable' sounded like 'a kitchen utensil'." Another reader joked about "getting one at the True Value Hardware."

In concluding, the word "disabled" won out over "handicapped." (Note: *The Disability Rag* has recently been renamed *The Ragged Edge*.)

Even the well-intentioned editor of a general-interest magazine made me wince with her subtitle for my article, "New York City on Wheels of Sorts." She added, "New York has it all. Getting to where it is, however, is not easy when you're confined to a wheelchair." True, when you are *"confined"* to a wheelchair, getting about is not easy. I mean, how do you take a bath or sleep at night under such circumstances? I transfer to a chair at a restaurant, to a seat at the movies, to a couch for relaxation. Most wheelchair users I know transfer to something, somewhere, at some time. In fact, I do not know anyone who stays in a wheelchair round the clock. Simply, wheelchairs — or any assistive device requiring long hours of sitting—are not that plush.

In the same vein, I am not *"afflicted."* Yech. What a horrible way to feel. Yes, I have multiple sclerosis, and too, I have other things — like a sense of caring, morality, spirituality and humor — to name a few. In other words, being "afflicted" or "tormented" by a disease is not really a part of my thinking, simply because there is so much more to life. Sure, I do not deny the illness, but I certainly do not feel "afflicted" by it. There is a big gap in thinking here.

"Sufferer?" Far from it. I don't suffer. Granted, life is a bit more difficult, but the suffering only occurs at certain times, like when I have a crackerjack headache. "Sufferer" is a noun. "To suffer" is a verb, an activity. It is not something I do all the time. But, I must confess, we all suffer on occasion, like when a headache occurs.

When referring to people who are deaf, saying "the deaf" is okay. The "deaf community" or the "deaf culture" are also appropriate. The "hard of hearing" appreciate being called just that as well. But neither the deaf nor the hard of hearing communities like "hearing-impaired," as it is considered too generic. The "hearing-disabled" is also considered questionable as a vague and euphemistic label. People appreciate that their specific hearing differences be known. The understood differences can guide others to appropriate means of communication.

Also, it goes without saying that blind people are people first. Remember the old adage: we are all linked in unity deeper than any difference. We are all people with individual characteristics. But our emotions are no different, sight or no sight. Our desires are no different, sight or no sight. To be a functional, contributing member of society is something we all wish. So, I recommend you say, using the person's name first, ". . . who is blind."

Yet, adjectives poorly placed are no better. Take this writer for example. Call me a "disabled writer" and I'd pout. Yes, I'd be a "disabled writer" if my computer were down. In fact, you would also pout under such circumstances. I would be happier, however, if you change things a bit by saying, "K.G. Stone, a writer with a disability . . ." Without thinking a lot about this, your language can improve images and attitudes tremendously. Too, it is so simple an act.

Since labeling is considered a provocative subject by many, it is certainly worth thinking about. Right now, you may feel confused and rather tongue-tied. I was too—until I thought about it. Exercising common sense is probably the best approach. In other words, avoid the labels, put the person first, and enjoy one another, regardless.

2

SEEING THE BARRIERS

You ask, "What can I do to be a more compassionate, helpful person when facing someone with a disability?" Well, a little awareness of the multitude of barriers persons with disabilities face is an enormous step toward understanding any disability. Being equipped with this knowledge is a wonderful way to begin. Furthermore, it helps if you understand that some of these barriers stand in front of the person who has a disability, and that other barriers are more between such a person and others.

Comprehending the challenges *anyone* faces should be attempted by *everyone,* disabled or not. Too, it is a way we can practice universal compassion. Barriers take many forms. They can be attitudinal, architectural, environmental, economic, communicative, or even intrinsic. Because of all this, you may be thinking, "My word, there are barriers *everywhere.*"

Yes, this is true. But, mere recognition of the problems is a big step in paving the way, all puns intended. And because disability is a universal experience, creating a barrier-free world eventually involves everyone. Too, creating a barrier-free world today immediately helps the infant in learning to walk, permits the UPS worker to easily deliver packages, allows one's elderly parent to have a safe visit, and readies the world for any situation to come. As a friend says, "Nobody can predict a surprise."

Attitudinal Barriers

One of the most pervasive—and insidious—barriers is attitudinal. It is sneaky, because we absorb societal mannerisms without clearly recognizing we are doing so. This is most obvious when we watch, if we can bring ourselves to it, the "Jerry Lewis Telethon," traditionally held on Labor Day weekend. Jerry Lewis displays a woeful image of children with muscular dystrophy. He fosters an attitude of pity, the logic being that if you feel sorry for these children you will send in a donation. So naturally, viewers assume that pity is the norm. Wrong. Very wrong.

The reality is that *no one* who has a disability wants to be pitied. "Piss on pity" is the battle cry of persons with disabilities heard around the world. While at an international disability conference in Vancouver, British Columbia, called Independence '92, I heard one of the keynote speakers talk about one aspect of the pity factor. Joshua Malinga, a disability activist from Zimbabwe, talked about how the concept of charity plays into the attitude of pity and just how distasteful it can be. He said that of course we alleviate our guilt when we send money to any charity organization. But, do we ever follow up on the charity's mode of operation? Most likely, no. For many of us, just sending the money is enough action on our part.

Many charity organizations, probably due to being overwhelmed more than anything else, often direct to group homes any moneys earmarked for persons with disabilities. Because these charity-managed group homes for persons with disabilities tend to operate like nursing homes here in the United States, they are breeding grounds for dependence, not independence.

Recognizing another worldwide battle cry among persons with disabilities, "Independence, not dependence," we realize the pity/charity route is not the right direction at all. Persons with disabilities want and need to live as freely as anyone else. So you can see how the pity factor unconsciously picked up from the "Jerry Lewis Telethon" and the like can actually work against us. In fact, Joseph Shapiro's best-selling, historic book on the disability movement here in the United States, called *No Pity* (1993, Random House), gives you an idea of how prevalent the no-pity philosophy is.

Paternalistic behavior goes hand-in-hand with pity—again a very insidious thing to watch and eliminate. This behavior is particularly present among the medical and mental-health professionals. Persons with disabilities encounter people in these professions frequently. Paternalistic modes of thought are often projected by these professionals. Educators, school counselors, social workers, or supervisors in the work environment are equally prone to behave the same way toward persons with disabilities.

It goes without saying that a paternalistic approach tends to rub any recipient's fur the wrong way. A person with a disability, who is already dealing with a myriad of challenges, tends to feel extraordinarily frustrated when encountering this unnecessary, and often what feels like derogatory, manner. Consequently, those with paternalistic mannerisms often get a frustrated response from the recipient, and tend to incorrectly identify that person as an angry, uncooperative individual. Such a poor interchange is very misleading and unproductive for everyone involved.

How do you eliminate these barriers such as pity and paternalism, attitudes that are often unconsciously learned and, for some, somewhat invisible? The most obvious answer is simply, do not pity anyone. And equally, do not talk down to anyone. After all, isn't it a universal desire to be treated as an equal—disabled or not, female or male, young or old, of an ethnic minority or not?

Architectural Barriers

When thinking of architectural barriers, we often think immediately of steps. It is quite obvious. But that has not always been the case. Let me tell you a couple of stories.

When I needed to retrofit my adobe house to make it wheelchair-accessible, I interviewed a number of potential contractors. Since this was in pre-ADA (Americans with Disabilities Act) days, I have to admit that awareness of any architectural barrier was pretty low then.

When discussing how to eliminate the front entrance step, the contractor interviewed said, "It's only two and a half inches, so why bother?" Sitting in my wheelchair, I told him to take a roll and promptly ended the interview.

Hindsight—as always—now tells me, he simply was not aware of this challenge, formidable and obvious as it was to me. This brought to mind how Ellen Harland—then a self-employed architect in Santa Fe and now still an architect, but currently employed by the federal government—raised the consciousness of her clients at an architectural seminar back in 1989 without saying a word or even introducing herself.

Registration for the event was in the carpeted hallway just outside the seminar room in one of Santa Fe's more elegant hotels. The nearby meeting room was partitioned off by a heavy set of glass French doors. Actually, a very innocuous setting, if you ask me. But it was also very Santa Fe (read that as a place full of barriers, since persons with disabilities theoretically do not exist there in the minds of many).

After the participants registered, Ellen requested each one to enter the nearby seminar room via the manual wheelchair that she provided. Seated in the chair, notebooks and clipboards in their laps, the first thing these participants tried to do was get the wheelchair rolling over the thick hallway carpet. Too thick. And too early in the morning. Those that did make it five feet over the plush carpet to the nearby French doors probably had two cups of coffee already and were endowed with sufficient adrenaline to do so. Yet, not all of us drink the caffeinated stuff. With books and clipboards sliding off their laps, these individuals simply could not open the heavy door while simultaneously trying to move their mired wheelchairs on the thick carpet. At this juncture, need I say more?

For those who experience any kind of challenge, accessibility can make the difference between a life of freedom and a life of restrictions and dependence. A place to live is one thing;

a place that promotes independence in daily living is another. Housing for people with disabilities is a big issue. It is an issue that can be found across the nation. So when talking about architectural barriers, I'll focus only on the most basic unit: our homes.

According to almost any independent living resource center across the country, finding accessible housing at reasonable cost is difficult at best. Low-cost rentals are necessary for a large portion of persons with disabilities, since a vast majority have limited incomes. In fact, the waiting list for subsidized housing anywhere is long.

So, in waiting for a place, what do we do? Join the ranks of homeless people while trying to find a barrier-free place to live? Live with our aging parents? Risk injury while being lifted up a step or two? Be in an environmentally sickening locale while searching for a better place? Live in a costly nursing home draining family or government finances simply because no other option exists? Sounds horrendous. Yet, it happens all the time.

Many developers and builders complain about increased costs in building accessible spaces. This is a hollow argument. According to an old but extensive 1987 cost estimate study issued by the Department of Housing and Urban Development (HUD), construction costs of accessible features in new buildings amounted to less than one percent of total costs. Interestingly, a newer (1993) study for HUD shows how easy it is to provide accessibility without adding any square footage to floor plans in new construction. What this reveals is our need to rethink how we deal with spatial relationships. In other words, there is plenty of room to break any long-standing tradition here.

Costs are relative, anyway. How much do today's builders spend on tinted glass, whirlpools, hot tubs, real marble in bathrooms, and real stone on kitchen counters? And what about those indoor grills, glass brick walls, brass tub fixtures? One percent more for added access? It is certainly a lot cheaper than time spent in a nursing home.

Accessible features, according to Concrete Change,[1] a network of people in Atlanta who want to see all housing barrier-free, include two ordinary, but essential, things we can do: make no-step entrances and be sure all doors are thirty-two inches wide or wider. "Two things. Two really simple things," says Eleanor Smith, Concrete Change founder.

When I traveled overseas to photograph and write about accessible and aesthetic homes in Scandinavia, I discovered the building codes requiring accessibility have been around so long there that such features have been rather taken for granted for some time. In their case, there is no special treatment. Try to look in Scandinavia for an example of an accessible and aesthetic home to photograph? Forget it. *All* recently built dwellings are quite accessible and appear rather normal.

And *everyone*, from children to grandparents, realizes the benefits of such housing, appropriately labeled "universal homes." Of course, accessible dwellings are also safer homes. There is less tripping because there are fewer steps, fewer sills, fewer floor level changes. Looking at safety issues in any kind of dwelling, statistics disclose that tripping and falling accidents cause many more deaths than emergencies and evacuations in fires and earthquakes. "To be exact, they cause six times more deaths," according to Clara Yoshida in her report, *Three Stage Housing for Old People*.[2]

Those saying that accessibility is too expensive, too institutional-appearing, or too difficult to design are perpetrating myths that need changing. Barrier-free homes are simply not "kneeling housing"—a snide reference that a *New York Times* writer made when comparing such housing to lift-equipped buses. Accessible, aesthetic, architecturally barrier-free homes are graceful spaces, spaces that allow for all kinds of people to live in them at all times.

Environmental Barriers

Many, many things in our environment create barriers. Some are natural, some are created by man. Of course, it goes without saying that nature's steep, soft, and rough terrain is difficult to encounter, no matter what shape you are in. Add ice or snow or too much water and you have even more woes.

Add smoke, new carpeting, any kind of fragrance, certain building materials, or ordinary household cleaning solvents, and you have a different set of barriers for certain individuals who are dealing with environmental illnesses/multiple chemical sensitivity (EI/MCS). In fact, when traveling to Scandinavia in 1989, I found allergies, which include environmental illness and multiple chemical sensitivity, as one of the five categories of disabilities defined there.

Harking back to the canaries that miners carried to warn of leaking gas, people with EI/MCS can be called canaries of the world. This modern-day disabling illness is a warning of what we are doing to ourselves and to our planet. But it is a shame that people, or canaries, should carry such a burden and suffer so much because of our wanton ways.

There is a lot that can set off people with EI/MCS, a lot of things we never notice or simply take for granted. Take a wood- or coal-burning stove two blocks away, take the glue used to laminate plywood in a building, or take the pleasant-smelling moisturizing lotion we use on a daily basis. They all can be harmful.

Perfume? Don't bother even trying a sample. A whiff that comes with your fashion magazine permeates the other letters in the mail, causing further anguish for those dealing with EI/MCS. Obviously, life for these individuals can get very complicated. The barriers can be anywhere.

Transportation Barriers

Transportation is a very difficult barrier faced by persons with disabilities because it is such a basic component in anyone's life. No transportation can mean no job out there, no visiting friends, no shopping, or no doing errands. A lack of transportation is very isolating. In this terrible situation, you can definitely say one is house-bound. In fact, this is a punishment often given out to people who do not necessarily warrant jail time nor warrant total freedom. Instead, they are prisoners in their own homes.

When I initially became disabled, I was house-bound for some time due to the lack of transportation. With help from the family, I was able to get my own converted van. I wrote about this experience and include the piece here, because it gives personal meaning to this particular barrier. Read it, and you will then understand just how liberating breaking such a barrier can be.

> The traffic is light as I drive down Corrales Road. The errands are a stop at the post office and the frame shop. It's as normal as you can get, except, of course, the celestial activity overhead. The sky moves a lot today, sun dodging and shadow casting with clouds illustrating the breeze. Flowering plum and pear trees are in full bloom, daffodils gathered at their bases. Heaven is both up, and down, and all around.
>
> A hawk soars. So do I. He crees. I cry. We are moved. We are moving. I feel extraordinarily ordinary, like all the folks in the other cars, doing errands, noticing spring. These things so little are enormously accomplishing, enormously freeing.
>
> To drive again, oh how understated, how wonderful. Now the static horizon I have watched for eight months and sixteen days becomes fluid and mutable while I drive to the post office and frame shop.
>
> These words are written in the spring of 1989, shortly after I drove my newly purchased converted van equipped with wheelchair access and hand controls. I was, with family help, able to buy my way to this freedom.
>
> Yet, I am not totally free. There are my disabled brothers and sisters with, perhaps, no family to help, no municipality to support barrier-free public transportation. My eight confined months can be for others, years, a life. I am disturbed by this thought.
>
> Automobile use is the greatest mode of transportation here in the United States. The structure of our society

depends largely on transportation. I am no exception. The structure of my life depends on such.

Like most of you, I need wheels in order to work, do shopping, attend Sunday morning's worship gathering. My doctor is not nearby and the post office is a little too far to walk, or shall we say in my case, roll.

Yet, the increasing pollution and traffic woes we face necessitates alternative solutions—soon. Too, I am equally responsible for today's muck, driving my new van any place I please or need.

This is not just the next generation's problem, but ours, today—now—this minute. The population bulge is currently in its forties. It goes without much explaining that as we become older, we drive less. Cities such as Portland, Oregon; Vancouver, British Columbia; and Boras, Sweden, are well aware of this concern for good public transportation and have addressed these needs with thought, foresight, and unexpected but pleasant results.

These places look toward mobility as a human right. It is not something for "them." It is for all of us. The transport systems in these places encompass, to name a few, the elderly, the disabled community, our students, the poor, our homeless, job seekers—and our earth.

Take the community of Boras in southeastern Sweden for example. Their transportation system experimented with "service route" busing, a system designed with extensive accessibility measures, including sufficient handrails, arm supports, level steps, lifts, or ramps to all stops and terminals. For the sight-impaired, larger signs and audible announcements were added. For the hard of hearing and deaf individuals, well-placed maps of all routes and stops provided assistance. In addition, proper planning and extensive marketing became component requirements.

The routes went near residential areas and other stops often used by elderly and disabled travelers, such as health-care centers, restaurant and service centers, shopping centers, and entertainment locations. Important features of the service route were short distances between stops and comfortable boarding and disembarking with lots of time allowed.

The pleasant surprise? Their ongoing, but separate, public transportation system saw a drop in users. According to the then director-general of the Swedish Board of Transport, Mr. Norrbom, "Due to the added comfort, security, and social togetherness supplied by this special service route, we realized an increased popularity and use by the general public."

As a result, everyone started using this system and it became the transportation system of Boras, the separate public transportation system eliminated due to faltering ridership.

As part of the change to a united public transport system, work centers and additional routes were added to the more desired service route line. On the average, the extra costs ran two to three percent of the total investment costs. These busses were purchased with the proper equipment, and thus the higher costs of retrofitting were eliminated. Good planning and foresight. Payback was rapid due to the elimination of a separate bus system. And the economic waves rippled further.

More members of the disabled community joined the work force. Looking at the larger picture, this adds to the community's economic well-being by the population's increased discretionary income and tax support. In other words, everyone benefits.

Everyone co-mingles. More riders, less cars, and less pollution. The hawk soars. So do I. He crees. I cry. We are moved. We are moving.

Economic Barriers

Little may we think that dollars and cents can be barriers, but they are. Definitely. Persons with disabilities often encounter the lack, sadly enough, of having enough money to buy their independence. To wit, not having money for wheels, any kind of wheels, means being rather stuck, no? Don't laugh. It is not only a teenage experience. This happens to persons with disabilities as well. Too often.

As of this writing, at least a third of the nation does not have medical insurance. As a result, many of us fork out a great deal of money for tools to assist in living any sort of healthy and independent lifestyle—or have no money at all to fork out. As a friend said when talking about no savings, "At this point, there is nothing between you and the big, bad wolves out there."

Further on in this book (Chapter 23) you will find a lot more on how these economic barriers function just about everywhere in our lives.

Communication Barriers

There are those of us who cannot see, talk, or hear very well or at all. By the very nature of such limitations, we encounter enormous barriers.

I had a roommate who was blind. As sensitive as I may be to individuals with such disabilities facing barriers, Brett had to patiently and consistently point out to me just how daunting my language was for him. Because I was not precise enough in my conversations, Brett did not always know what I was talking about. To wit, when asking for the book "over there," I should be saying, "the book on the top of the shelf by the phone, three feet to your right." This may seem somewhat obvious, but for many of us, our method of communicating with blind individuals is rather unseeing in itself.

Communicating precisely is required even in the seeing world. I remember when working as a marketing professional for a large architectural-engineering firm, the staff would constantly ask me for more details. And currently, accuracy is an utmost requirement in my work as a writer. So, in conversing with, or writing to, any individual, any place, being more precise is a way of knocking down all sorts of barriers.

When it comes to one form of communicating, specifically that of talking, computers are now smashing the barriers more and more. Stephen Hawking, often referred to as "the best-known modern physicist since Einstein," author of *A Brief History of Time* and *Black Holes and Baby Universes and Other Essays*, lecturer, father, subject of a movie, is a person dealing with ALS, a degenerative nerve disease. This very brilliant individual now uses a voice synthesizer and additional computer technology in order to work and communicate. In his introduction to *Computer Resources for People with Disabilities*, Hawking writes:

> This book is about problems of expression and communication, and how to solve them. I am dumb, in the literal sense of not being able to speak. Maybe I'm dumb in the more figurative sense, but we won't go into that here. I, and thousands like me, have been helped to communicate by modern technology. Indeed, the fact that I have been asked to write this foreword is a sign of what technology can do. . . I hope others find in this book the inspiration and the technology, hardware and software, that can help them to communicate better—to express their human-ness.[3]

Hawking touches on a very important aspect of this modern technology. Go ahead and take advantage of its assistive power, but don't lose sight of the human being behind it. In other words, I may use this technological wonder, my computer, to communicate what I can in writing, but like you, I also cry, giggle, wonder how my neighbor is doing, and am in the process of planning tonight's meal.

Myths as Barriers

Certain myths or common beliefs about disability can create barriers that we might never think of as impeding a person relating to someone with a disability. But these beliefs can cause apathetic behavior, lack of knowledge, or even social ineffectiveness. Perhaps the following long letter I wrote to a young friend back in 1990 will help explain how this can be.

Dear Jeffrey,

You know someone who now uses a wheelchair, someone with whom you previously hiked, raced up stairs at school, and played softball together. As a result of a car accident, your friend, Sean, is "a para, a wheelie," so we crips say to one another. Oh, what do you say? What do you do, now?

Sean, your friend, is now dealing with paraplegia, is now a wheelchair user. Nothing new, yet everything new. But, no surprise. A well-known fact is that teenagers are one of the largest groups of people with disabilities who end up using wheelchairs due to accident.

Jeffrey, I understand your feeling awkward and agonizing over "the accident." You have not seen Sean for a year, you're attending different colleges. Jeffrey, you want to visit so much, but what to say? How to reconnect? How to behave?

Granted it takes courage to look at someone who can no longer do these things with you now, to look at someone who appears less capable (in your eyes), to look at someone who may, in fact, actually be more dependent in some ways and have a different set of needs. Oh, what to say? How to behave?

Before I answer "What do I say? What do I do?" let me step into Sean's world for a minute and explain some of what he is going through right now. Dispelling the notion that those of us with disabilities idly sit at home,

I need to explain to you, Jeffrey, just how time-consuming the transition, the adjustments, the learning how to cope can be. In brief, Sean is obtaining a Ph.D. in life.

Jeffrey, we were not raised as very emotionally honest people. If anything, we tend to run away from "the tragedies of life." It is indeed scary—to look at what very well may happen to any one of us, anytime. We tend to think of this as the end of life. I cannot tell you how many people have said, "Karen, I don't know how you do (did) it. I couldn't." To which I have always answered, "You simply do it. You cross that bridge when it's there for you to cross."

Sean is now doing the crossing. And at times, he probably is tired, frustrated, angry, and grieving. We've all experienced some of these feelings. To face them all at once is indeed scary. As you know from your own experience, not much can be done about this roller-coaster trip, other than to acknowledge, accept, and ride it out, all puns intended. And let time proffer us the badly needed patience here.

In addition, getting this kind of Ph.D. requires multi-level skills: psychological, physical, emotional—to be utilized simultaneously and with phenomenal intensity. Stall and you might stumble. Procrastinate and you might stultify. Go too fast and you might run out of gas. So how can you help someone here?

Help? Do you need to try to help? Can you just be yourself? Can you just hang out instead? As always in the past, your friends have brought you stories, gossip, jokes, and more of the same ol' stuff. There is a sense of continuum in so simple an act. For Sean, it is a break from the intense Ph.D. work. A point of relaxation. A crap shoot. Small, significant, and wonderful.

So, Jeffrey, what do you say? Nothing but the same old stuff. Sure, you ask Sean if he would like help. You did that as high school buddies, and as before, Sean is free to say yea or nay. Sure, you talk about your own vulnerabilities and acknowledge your awkwardness. You did that before, too.

Sure, Sean is not standing as tall, so you plop down into an easy chair to be on equal eye level when conversing together. Sure, you "run along" when doing errands together. That is what you did—and said—before the accident.

Sure, you horse about like you used to, arm wrestling fist to table. The contact is something you previously did. Granted, you are both over six feet tall, and to date, you have never patted Sean on the head. You don't start that now. It would be a patronizing and demeaning gesture at best. Likewise, you do not lean on Sean's wheelchair, because that is part of his personal body space.

And when you are both out with buddies, friends should equally rap to Sean, and not rap to him via you. Sean can still see, hear, exercise judgment, and talk. He may ask one of you for directions, simply because you're taller, and in that regard, a scout of sorts. But, he is, in final analysis, still the expert in getting himself about, not you.

"Isolation is almost as debilitating as the disability itself," says peer counselor Carlos Diaz. Because of existing physical and attitudinal barriers, it is harder for persons with disabilities to mingle. Break that. Explore what you can do together. Scout ahead. And make sure it is an activity that you do on equal footing. In other words, make sure the access is there. For those of us in wheelchairs, we dislike, to mildly state, "being lifted up the one four-inch step that is in the way." Though only four inches, it simply is not equal footing.

All you need to remember, Jeffrey, is simply to be you, nothing more, nothing less. After all, when I became a wheelie, I never said anything different to you.

Some of the myths about persons with disabilities are quite prevalent, reflecting the incorrect thinking of many. The good news is that in just becoming aware of these myths, you move toward realizing how limiting these misconceptions can be.

"Awareness is the first step towards change," according to the National Easter Seal Society.

But myths are very difficult to dispel. Says Jim Byrnes, actor and disability rights activist, "When I lost my legs in an accident almost twenty years ago, it never occurred to me that one of my biggest problems would be how people reacted to my disability."

I have not only run into this problem a number of times, but have experienced a multitude of other misconceptions as well. In fact, one person came up to me and asked, "What's wrong with you?" Out of both patience and humor, I responded by wryly saying, "And what is right about you?"

One of the most prevalent myths is that people with disabilities don't want to, or cannot, work. The fact is that, according to numerous polls taken over the years, persons with disabilities want the same opportunities to pursue careers and support themselves or their families as anyone else. Two-thirds of all adults with disabilities are unemployed while a very large percentage of this group wish to work. Many persons with disabilities are educated, talented, and qualified to work.

Adapting workplaces for persons with disabilities often costs far less than people think. On the average, these costs run $500 or less, according to Job Accommodation Network. In fact, providing accommodation costs far less than the billions of dollars we spend on things such as unemployment or the military.

Take, for example, two articles on facing pages in the July 8, 1992 issue of a local newspaper, the *Albuquerque Journal*. One headline said "Disabilities Act Remodeling Costs to Pass $2 Million" (for the entire state of New Mexico). On the opposite page, a smaller headline claimed, "Sandia [Laboratories] Repairs to Cost $200 Million." Such headlines perpetuate the myth that accommodating persons with disabilities in the work environment is too costly.

There is an abundance of misconceptions. The National Easter Seal Society points out a more few common myths and illusions:

- **MYTH:** Persons with disabilities live vastly different lives than most people.

  Fact: Many persons with disabilities need to do the laundry, shop for food, get gas for their vehicle, pay bills, worry about the kids, buy or build homes, work in the garden, get involved in political activities or indulge in a tasty dessert, just as you and I do.

- **MYTH:** Persons with disabilities are brave and courageous.

  Fact: Adjustment to a disability involves adaptation to a total lifestyle change rather than being courageous or brave. We did not choose to become disabled nor did we resolve to become brave. Simply, we have decided to adapt and carry on.

- **MYTH:** Persons with disabilities are more at ease with "their own kind."

  Fact: With the seasoned independent living movement and the passage of the ADA, you have seen or will find more and more persons with disabilities involved with all kinds of people in mainstream activities.

- **MYTH:** Wheelchair use is "confining" or users of wheelchairs are "wheelchair bound."

  Fact: We are not "bound" or "confined" to the wheelchair. We transfer out of the chair to take a shower, to go to bed, to listen to a concert—like glasses, wheelchairs are merely personal assistive devices. Just think of what life would be without these tools.

- **MYTH:** Persons with disabilities always need help.

  Fact: Yes, help may be needed at times, but not at all times. Many persons with disabilities are independent, are quite willing—and want—to give help themselves. Also, the more our environment becomes accessible, the less helpless one may be.

• **MYTH:** Children should never ask persons about their disability.

  Fact: Let's face it, children are naturally curious. Parents tend to get embarrassed when their child starts asking questions. However, most persons with disabilities do not mind this. And, in trying to prevent children from asking questions, adults try to hide or stop their child's curiosity, actually giving these youngsters the impression that there is something bad about disabilities.

Inger Nordqvist of Sweden says, "Work to eliminate myths such as 'There is something strange about someone who marries a disabled person.' Or about single mothers—'How can she, who has a [disabled] boy/girl, go out and have a good time?'"

Myths do proliferate and are a challenge to allay. The disability community at large is doing its best to dispel these myths and stereotypes. Trying to be more aware of your own assumptions helps a great deal. This awareness helps you overcome any apathetic mannerisms. In doing so, a wonderful thing happens. Your heightened awareness will make your connections with persons with disabilities that much more enjoyable and graceful.

Just keep in mind that if we, persons with disabilities, seem somewhat impatient in our reply to you, it is simply because we have explained these things over and over again to others. Plus, we are simultaneously dealing with a lot of other obstacles and challenges. I am sure you have an inkling by now. This is where your compassionate understanding, not pity, comes into play.

Still nervous? Tell a good joke. Bring some fabulous food. Gossip. Be yourself. Cry, if necessary. Share. Laugh together. But most important, be genuine.

3

INVISIBLE
DISABILITIES

There is a plethora of disabilities, some obviously visible, some not, some coming with birth, some acquired later on. Whether visible or acquired early on in life, whether invisible or acquired later on, having a disability undoubtedly colors one's life.

No one is an expert about the vast variety of possible disabilities, yours truly included. It is impossible to become an expert in all. However, almost everyone can be candid, frank, and honest in their interaction with others, thereby becoming an expert in learning—which, fortunately, is a never-ending process in our lives. To wit, when encountering the unknown, I openly say, "I don't know much about your condition. Can you explain a little to me?" To date, I've yet met anyone who has had trouble with this honest, straightforward approach. After all, I am asking the best expert in this specific case.

On the other hand, I've encountered those who have had difficulty relating to me because of my disability, so unfortunately, the ball is in my court to respond first. The need is pretty obvious. I can see it in their nervous eyes. I say, "unfortunately," because this is still the case more often than not. Once again, no matter how tired I may be, I have to dredge up additional patience and humor so I can put this person at ease.

I do this by saying, "You are probably wondering why I use this motorized rickshaw. It is because . . ." and the conversation unfolds. I give the person permission to ask questions—as many as they may have. "It's absolutely okay," I reiterate, "anytime." Putting others at ease in this manner works like magic. People are curious, so it is most gracious to allow for such. On the other hand, silence and ignorance hurts everyone, over time.

Invisible disabilities include a myriad of conditions. There are those of us who have learning or developmental difficulties, a hearing loss, environmental sensitivities, asthma, brain injuries, arthritis, and more, much more. The list goes on. Invisible disabilities are widespread. It is ironic that conditions so prevalent should be called "invisible." We are a lot more surrounded by invisible disabilities than anyone realizes.

Brain Injury

Take head injury. Unobvious as it may be, we probably all know someone with a brain injury. From something as simple as a fall to a more traumatic accident, from a whiplash to a stroke, from an uncanny illness to a difficult birth, a large number of individuals have encountered some kind of insult to their brain. A very large number.

And the extent of the injuries is immense, ranging from an innocuous whiplash to deep coma. According to the National Head Injury Foundation, 700 thousand persons per year in the United States alone receive some kind of head injury. Each year 100 thousand persons die from such injury and an estimated 70 to 90 thousand are permanently disabled. What these figures do not represent are those who receive a mild blow to the head and do not get follow-up treatment, unaware that there may have been some injury to the brain.

Months later, job difficulties may arise because of the insult to the head that has occurred with a seemingly harmless blow. This is surprisingly common, more common than we think.

Also, brain injury is a challenge for the medical professional, partner, friend, boss, co-worker and/or child, let alone the one with the actual brain trauma. The coping skills, memory retention, and community activities of the affected individual are wounded as well. It is not that these people are "mentally retarded" as some are mistakenly identified, but simply, that their brains are both insulted and trapped by injury.

I asked a doctor who specializes in the field of traumatic brain injury how it might be most helpful to interact with a brain-injured individual. There are numerous approaches, obviously too many to discuss here. However, he did mention one thing in brief, addressing a very common problem that often occurs when interacting with a brain-injured person. When asking a question that might lead to further confusion, simply restate the question in a different way. Oh, how true this can be in a variety of situations. We find that this is the best thing to do with our children, an elderly parent, an individual with a hearing loss, or a perplexed coworker. In other words, regardless of the person you are with, it is most useful to express some ingenuity and patience.

Hearing Loss and Deafness

Most likely we all know someone with a hearing loss. According to one certified audiologist I know, roughly ten percent of Americans have some degree of hearing loss, including yours truly.

Around those who have a hearing loss, we tend automatically to speak louder. Many times, this is not necessary. There are those of us who wear hearing aids, and a louder voice actually distorts what is being said. Once again, a simple rephrasing of the comment or question is all that is warranted. Also, covering your mouth while you are talking makes it difficult for another to read your lips. And you would be surprised how often that occurs. Too, we all have been at a party with loud noise in the background where it was difficult for *anyone* to hear.

"It is not what you don't hear, but it's what is in between the ears" says Robert Geesey, an executive director on the Commission for the Deaf and Hard of Hearing in New Mexico. The deaf community is a community that is being heard more and more. Take the news programs on TV. Closed captioning for most programs is now a standard across the nation. Take the telephone relay networks. They allow a hearing person to converse easily with a deaf person on the phone by use of a telecommunication display device (TDD). A hearing operator at a relay network station will type in your comment for the deaf individual to read on the TDD unit. And vice versa. Use of these networks is getting to be a commonplace practice. And then, there is e-mail . . .

So what can you, the hearing person, do in the actual presence of deaf people, especially if you don't know sign language?

- If there is advance notice that a deaf person is coming to your event, make sure there is an interpreter in attendance. Ask if the deaf person is bringing someone or if you must hire an interpreter.

- If an interpreter is present, address the person you are conversing *with,* not the interpreter. The same applies to those who are using the phone relay system. The intermediate relay operator, like the interpreter, is simply a tool for communicating.

- If no interpreter is on hand, speak slowly, and mouth the words distinctly so that lips may be read. It is imperative that hands do not cover the speaker's mouth, something one might do when casually sitting and relaxing. Also, note that bushy mustaches sometimes make lip reading difficult.

- Watch your lighting. The lip reader will have trouble reading if the light source is behind you. The reader primarily sees you in silhouette, while your lips are in shadow.

- Among the deaf, to scream is pointless and considered a no-no. It is embarrassing. In such a situation, all communication is lost. It is best to simply mouth the words well. In fact, Geesey says, "I know people who mouth words silently."

- At last resort, you can write notes. It is awkward in a group, but works fine in a one-to-one situation.

Sure, the deaf person needs to look at the interpreter and not at you while conversing. Sure, phone conversations lack the normally heard tonal expressions because of the intermediate relay operator. Sure, writing out a conversation can be slow. But you are doing something very important. You are communicating with one another, and in doing so, you are bridging the gap.

Environmental Illness

Another invisible disability involves environmental illness, a sensitivity or allergy to many man-made products. So rampant is this condition that it is fully acknowledged, recognized, and categorized as a disabling condition in Scandinavia. This allergy is one of the five categories of disability defined there.

Joan Sullivan-Cowan of Albuquerque, New Mexico, and a person very aggravated by environmental illness/multiple chemical sensitivity (EI/MCS), reminds us of something she read in Rachel Carson's classic book, *Silent Spring*, first published in 1962. Joan asked back in 1993, "As we remember the Holocaust . . . will we realize that the chemicals used in the 'gassing rooms' were really pesticides? The deadly nerve gas, Zyklon B, is an organic ester of phosphoric acid."

There are those of us who get a crackerjack headache at the mere whiff of a new carpet in our office, those of us who find a woman's perfume triggering a severe allergic reaction, and those of us whose esophagus almost swells shut in the presence of smoke drifting down from our chimneys.

What has started me thinking about all this these days is the strange commonality certain ailments share, such as all kinds of cancer, chronic fatigue syndrome, environmental illness/multiple chemical sensitivity, multiple sclerosis, and a host of other mysterious and disabling ailments.

Back in 1992, I wrote: "The obscure Gulf War syndrome should be added. Largely, all are conditions caused by the unknown—or should I say, 'known, but unspoken' causes? However, toxic chemicals are suspect in every case." Interestingly, as of this writing, independent studies are contradicting the FBI reports that claim there is "absolutely no physiological basis for the Gulf War Syndrome." Yet, the independent studies are saying that Gulf War survivors are now dealing with permanent neurological damage caused precisely by their exposure to pesticides used there.

No surprise. Even years ago, in 1989, the Environmental Protection Agency was reporting that:

- Ninety-nine percent of the population has one or more toxic chemicals stored in their fatty tissue.

- Ninety-five percent of all mothers' milk is toxic from pesticides found in our food, water, and homes.

And then, in the same year, the National Cancer Institute was saying:

- Over one out of three of us will have cancer.

- Ninety-eight percent of all cancer is caused by toxic chemicals.

And the National Academy of Sciences in Air Pollutants estimated in 1981 that up to fifteen percent of the United States population suffer from chemical sensitivities. I believe this figure is much higher today. People with EI/MCS react in varying degrees to manmade agents such as solvents, fragrances, drugs, cosmetics, auto/industrial emissions, pesticides, herbicides—anycide for that matter—and a host of other agents. These allergic-like reactions to man-made toxins often can result in neurological damage. Or cancer. Or death. Such reactions are largely triggered by the pollutants that so permeate our world. Needless to say, there is a jungle of hazardous chemicals to those with EI/MCS, no matter how clean the environment. In fact, even cleaning agents can give someone with EI/MCS an acute and damaging, if not fatal, reaction.

Just who gets EI/MCS? Almost anyone. Anytime. Some people merely need one exposure to a sensitizing agent to trigger this condition (for example, an insecticide mixture) while others become ill only after repeated exposures (such as a dry cleaning plant worker).

Mental Illness

One of the least understood and often most ignored invisible disabilities is mental illness. Says one social worker in the field, "I believe society will learn to accept physical, sensory, and learning disabilities. This will happen long before mentally related disabilities are dealt with." And the National Alliance for the Mentally Ill, a self-help organization that also includes family and friends as members, finds the most shocking thing about mental illness to be "how little people understand it."

The mentally ill community has been given a poor image because of a few notorious people who have been infamous for their horrible deeds and consequently have received much publicity. They are often categorized as "totally insane." Perhaps so, but there is also a vast number of mentally ill individuals who do not fall into this category. So in this case, it's very important to separate the trees from the forest.

Mental illness does not mean mental retardation. The former primarily involves moods, not intelligence. Mental retardation means a diminished intelligence, usually present at birth, and usually caused by some trauma during pregnancy or at birth, such as drinking alcohol during pregnancy or poor delivery techniques.

Mental illness, on the other hand, can affect persons at any age. It can result in disturbances in thinking, feeling, or the ability to relate to others. And it can substantially diminish one's capacity for coping with daily activities and life in general. Some categories of mental illness include schizophrenia, bipolar illness (manic-depressive illness), autism, seasonal affective disorder, and various forms of depression. Other conditions can include intense abuse of alcohol and drugs, extreme anxiety, and personality or behavioral disorders. With any of these conditions, you are not "insane." You are ill.

The causes of mental illnesses are not very well understood. Currently, it is believed that the brain's neurotransmitters are involved. There are many factors that may contribute to the onset, such as stress, recreational drugs, or heredity. Unfortunately, mental illnesses are misdiagnosed many times. A doctor can be fooled by the patient's behavior, failing to realize that an underlying physical cause can actually be the source of the problem.

As of late, however, there has been a great deal of research, some of it conclusive, into the links connecting mental illness to nutrition and mental illness to physical ailments. Such distinctive exploration is most encouraging. And, I believe, a step in the right direction. Since many illnesses, such as heart disease, diabetes, or colitis, are believed to have an origin in dietary causes, it is a logical step to think that there may be a similar dietary/nutritional link to mental illnesses.

Research suggests an increased likelihood that there is a significant relationship. As a result, there is a further refinement of feasible nutritional approaches to solving such problems. However, a word of caution. In this case, there is simply no way we can self-diagnose or self-treat. Mental conditions are extremely complex and hard to understand, so the input of those with a Ph.D. in chemistry or biology often is required.

Do you remember what Marilyn Monroe often told photographers when they would comment on her beauty? She would say to them, "You always take pictures of my body, but my most perfect features are my teeth—I have no cavities." Well, research now tells us that people under study, who salivated easily, had few cavities. Too, people who salivated easily often had a high histamine level in their body. People with this high histamine level would often be depressed and suicidal as well. This grim reaper may have taken the lives of Marilyn Monroe, Judy Garland, and Shane O'Neill (the son of Eugene O'Neill). The constant threat of suicide is one of the greatest problems found in people with an unusually high histamine levels. Part of a whole regimen of treating high histamine levels involves reducing the intake of folic acid. And those of us who take megadoses of multivitamins risk changing the folic acid balance in our bodies with such a practice.

This makes me think, is there a possible connection between teen suicides and their histamine levels? Are today's teen dietary habits responsible for raising their histamine levels?

Of course, I do not know. But what I do know is that proper nutrition plays a big role in my own personal mental well-being. A few years back, out of the blue, I started getting panic attacks. They were devastating, very frightening, and uncontrollable. With no warning, they would randomly occur on any given day, but always in the early evenings. (And I wasn't afraid of the dark, even as a child.)

To make a long story short, it turned out to be a protein deficiency, the result of my being a vegetarian and primarily eating only large salads for midday meals. The attacks promptly ended when I started to increase my protein intake by consuming nuts around four in the afternoon. This experience not only underscores the value of good nutrition in our lives for our mental well-being, it also underscores the need of working with a knowledgeable professional. Granted, my helper did not have a Ph.D. in nutrition, but he had a Ph.D. in psychiatry and then some. And he practices holistic healing—in other words, he heals the whole person, not just the mind.

Remember the movie, *King of Hearts*, with Alan Bates? This wonderfully zany film takes place in a small French village abandoned during World War II. Residents of a local "insane asylum" find their place left unlocked. The heart of the story involves their exploration of the outside world until the Nazis arrive to invade the place. When the military enters, they find a surprise awaiting them. Then the theme of the movie becomes obvious: who is *really* off balance? The film poses a very good question, a question treated with delightful humor and good taste. Who really is to judge?

When I lived in a small town in the foothills of northern California, there were eighty of us who lived there, including one—but probably others as well—who was and is developmentally disabled. She was and is protected by her close neighbors and family living nearby. She has her own house, a place the family owns and maintains. She lives alone, everyone checking in on her; she checking in on everyone. Since leaving that place, I realize I miss her daily singsong greeting, "Hi, Karen, how are you?" as I walked to the post office. My answer did not really matter. It was the ritual that mattered.

Because this town is situated in the Gold Rush country of California, there are bits of remnant evidence of miner activity to be found in the oddest places when taking a walk in the surrounding forested hills and valleys. You suddenly come upon a black walnut or mission fig tree, still standing at a place where once a log house stood. The population of this place was more than ten times its current size during the town's heyday in the mid-1800s gold rush.

So there she would be, calling out with her singsong "Hi, Karen" and snapping me back into reality as I wandered to the post office. If I was lucky, she would treat me to a bucket of fresh blackberries picked earlier in the coolness of that morning. But most of the time, we would hire her to pick berries for us or to crack the harvested and dried walnuts found in the backwoods that were supposedly wild and certainly organic. What a treat—those fresh, organic black walnuts.

She is now sixty-five, and probably still blessing folks with her greetings and blackberries. I always took her presence for granted. I grew up with her being a part of town. I always knew she was developmentally disabled. So? That I respected and treated her like any one of us was a normal facet of my life there, of my exchange with her. This experience gave me a lifelong understanding and acceptance of our differences. Given the right set of circumstances, I realize that different folks of all sorts can be great neighbors. As in *King of Hearts*, the line between "us" and "them," between the so-called "sane" and "insane," remains fuzzy. Who is to really judge?

Setting these questions aside for a moment, is it not the responsibility of those who live in the outside (read that as outside of an institution) to help keep others in the mainstream of our lives? Forget the professionals and government for a moment. Ask yourself what you can do, even if it seems so trite, so insignificant. Is not life a sum of small parts anyway?

Depression

Much as we would like to sweep the topic under the rug, the reality of depression is very present among an untold number of people, including both the affected persons and their surrounding folks. And they say depression goes with the territory of being, or becoming, disabled.

But what about people who are homeless or people who have been abused or people who are recovering from some kind of trauma? Exactly whose territory are we talking about when it comes to depression? Actually, it takes very little looking or sensitivity to realize that someone around us is depressed. And it can be very important to realize it.

Although I am reputed to be a no-quitter, I once called it quits. Believing there was gospel truth in the saying, "I'd rather be dead than disabled," I attempted suicide. Getting physically worse, resigning from my job, becoming financially insecure, ending a long-term relationship, trying to adjust, needing time to relate to all the changes, and more, simply overwhelmed me. Depressed? Yes, I'd say so.

Could my sense of helplessness and hopelessness have been averted? By anyone? By anything? Maybe so, maybe not. Had I a wheelchair-accessible place to go, to rest, to comfortably "chill out" from the crises so to speak, I might not have taken such drastic action. And to be able simply to talk with someone aware and sensitive to disability challenges might have given me a greater sense of order and continuum. Too, I really needed to be reassured that there definitely was life after a wheelchair.

But because it was still the days before the ADA (Americans with Disabilities Act), the world around me felt largely *inaccessible*. I felt trapped, helpless, and hopeless. Where could I go? Who could I see? How could I carry on? Sadly, many people with disabilities continue to feel the same today—and with good reason. Our society primarily revolves around activities of an able-bodied society. For the nondisabled, this can mean merely hopping into the car to go to the gym for a good workout or to see a therapist whose office is up four steps—simple as that. Due to inaccessibility, people with disabilities are required to live the "special, but separate" life. In other words, we are rather isolated.

How depressing. When you see this kind of isolation, it is important to stay in touch with a person who may be depressed, who may be confounded by what appear to be overwhelming obstacles. At a time like this, it's the small things that count, like taking a walk outdoors. Sharing. The sun, cold air, a bit of exercise, and time together can offer a stimulating and very needed moment. But think about where you do go. Make sure it is a quiet space. John Burroughs once said, "I go to Nature to be soothed and healed, and to have my senses put in tune once more."

Just make sure you and the person dealing with depression have plenty of these moments together. Hard as it may be, stay connected. This can be lifesaving. Depression is, at times, most devastating. I can attest to this based on personal experience. You cannot solve this person's problems. Don't even try. Just be your everyday self. Be human. Be open. Be powerfully honest. And says Cynthia Sontag, a licensed independent social worker, "Empower the individual. Allow them to make their own choices and be as neutral as possible. Do your job as a friend and let the professionals treat the depression."

For years, there has been a great deal of discussion, writing, debating, and theorizing about depression. You would think that by now we would have more of a handle on it, with all the research, money, and effort being put into this particular illness. But in fact, we still know very little and are still very baffled by its causes.

William Styron, author of *Sophie's Choice*, *The Confessions of Nat Turner*, and other novels, writes eloquently about his own depression in *Darkness Visible: A Memoir of Madness* (Random House, 1990). It is a book I highly recommend for anyone and everyone. An excellent read, it is short, to the point, insightful, quite revealing, and very powerful.

Styron spends a fair amount of time writing about depression as a disease and one of its possible, and frequent, manifestations, suicide. He reports that up to twenty percent of depressed individuals take their lives. Styron talks quite frankly about the number of suicides and the impulse toward it among individuals dealing with depression. He says, "The pain of severe depression is quite unimaginable to those who have not suffered it, and it kills in many instances because its anguish can no longer be borne."

Styron lights into those who seem mystified about why anyone would take their life, without taking into consideration the struggle one endures while dealing with the overwhelming impact of depression. He states that the post-suicide/attempt guessing game by others probably creates more damage than understanding as to why anyone would self-destruct. Styron comments on "the number of people for whom the subject [suicide] had been taboo, a matter of secrecy and shame." In reading Styron's memoir, I now understand more clearly how down I was, low enough to be compelled to self-destruct. How strange a period for me.

Basically, I am a person of deep spirit, of a strong love for life, light, and compassion.

Styron, too, survived his ordeal. He concludes by saying, ". . . men and women who have recovered from the disease — and they are countless — bear witness to what is probably its [depression's] only saving grace: it is conquerable." But in this lucidly written and well-researched memoir, Styron reminds us, "Depression is much too complex in its cause, its symptoms and its treatment, for unqualified conclusions to be drawn from the experience of a single individual."

In retrospect, I'm glad my attempt failed. The recovery was long, slow, and painful. But, the problem was conquerable. Granted, it gave me a few gray hairs, yet it resulted in some amazing insight and growth, to say at the least. It is sad that others do not have this opportunity to look back, to recognize that the attempt was a hopeless, and oh so unnecessary, act.

More than ever, at a time of depression, we need to remain in touch with others. Yes, like most human beings, I still have my bouts with doubts, but now I have a support system that makes sure my life raft stays afloat. Too, I have hope, heightened by all the warm hearts surrounding me. I have compassion, widened by understanding. I have understanding, expanded by experience. I have life, deepened by the closeness of death.

Seasonal Affective Disorders

Most of us do not care for the standard time change that occurs in winter, with our outdoors activities cut short by darker days and inclement weather. We feel more lethargic, have less energy, want to sleep longer or eat more. It is no wonder that some of us shrink at the thought of turning our clocks back. In fact, some of us get downright depressed during the winter months.

The annual rhythm of getting depressed in the winter darkness is often referred to as seasonal affective disorder (SAD). This condition is far more widespread than most of us believe.

In fact, it is estimated by researchers that 10 million of the United States population suffer from SAD, and an additional 25 million endure a milder form of the condition known as the "winter blues" or "winter blahs." SAD is a recurring condition. It involves mood and behavior changes so powerful in the winter months that its impact can produce significant problems in our lives. The more common "winter blues" however, involve some lesser degree of seasonal change for most. Energy levels, sleeping patterns, eating habits, and mood can vary.

Do you have SAD? Dr. Norman Rosenthal, a pioneer in research on SAD and author of the book, *Seasons of the Mind* (Bantam, 1989), has designed a questionnaire to help people discover if they have SAD. As to its cause, Dr. Rosenthal theorizes that the pineal gland in the brain releases a hormone called melatonin when the body experiences long periods of darkness. The melatonin can cause adverse emotional effects. Bright light, on the other hand, suppresses the secretion of melatonin.

Most people with SAD are women. The onset of the condition often occurs in their early twenties. But many people with SAD report a marked improvement with any change involving climate, latitude, and light conditions—in other words, relocating to sunny and warmer locales. Similarly, people with SAD respond favorably to an improvement in the weather or to being moved from a windowless office to one with a window. Conversely, deterioration in mood and energy levels often occurs when the amount of environmental light is reduced.

More and more professionals in the mental health field are treating people for this very real phenomenon. It is considered a serious, but treatable, disorder. The common method of therapy today is light treatment (photo therapy). Though only recently utilized, photo therapy has a history. As far back as 1845, a Dr. Esquirol described a patient with a syndrome resembling SAD. He effectively treated this person by recommending that he winter in sunny Italy instead of remaining in the darker winter days of Belgium.

However, the existence of photo therapy doesn't mean you should race out and buy light bulbs with higher wattage. Photo therapy involves a very specific prescription: so much illumination, for so long, and with certain types of light bulbs. Possible side effects, though uncommon, can include irritability, eyestrain, headaches or insomnia: thus the importance of getting treatment with an experienced professional.

Light obviously plays an enormous factor in our lives. It is no surprise that drinking and suicides in Scandinavia increase during their dark winter days. It is also no surprise that most of us anticipate the "spring forward" phenomenon that comes with changing our clocks again.

I have a lot of windows and skylights in this small adobe home of mine. In fact, as I sit here and write this, I look out of the enormous windows behind my computer. I can see the sky and variable weather patterns. I watch the light changing on the mountains at different times of the day. I witness trees turning color and crows batting about, this being their playfield during the winter months. And as I look out, the incoming light lowers my melatonin. What a blessing.

In concluding, though there may be no cure for many mental illnesses, depression included, there is a wide range of medications and therapy can that help to reduce symptoms a great deal. In some cases, symptoms are so successfully reduced that an individual, with the support of a good family and community program, can live independently, work, get married, and have children.

Developmental Disabilities

Other common invisible conditions include a range of developmental disabilities, often caused by a birth trauma or a brain injury of a youngster or even lead poisoning. There is also growing evidence of the connection between alcohol consumption by pregnant women and the resulting mental retardation of newborns, often referred to as the fetal alcohol syndrome. Some additional examples of the invisible developmental disabilities include epilepsy, autism, communicative disorders, chromosomal disorders, cerebral palsy, and seizure disorders.

Fetal Alcohol Syndrome

Being exposed to the alcohol the mother drinks during pregnancy puts an unborn child at risk for a myriad of lifelong difficulties. For the mother's pleasure of untimely drinks, the fetus can be affected. It's a lousy trade-off. With what is commonly known as fetal alcohol syndrome (FAS), the affected child can be born with all kinds of behavioral difficulties, learning challenges, mental retardation, or other health problems.

What FAS statistics exist are disturbing. According to a Center for Substance Abuse Prevention 1993 technical report, "It has been estimated that five to eleven percent of all pregnant women drink at levels that may place their infants at risk, and that up to thirty percent of infants born to women who are heavy drinkers exhibit signs of FAS or fetal alcohol effects (FAE)." In fact, according to numerous resources, FAS is the leading known cause of mental retardation. Also, FAS babies are at greater risk for infant mortality. Is that what you want to give to your child, to any child, to society?

FAS costs the nation untold dollars. The price is staggering. We pay taxes to provide special education programs for those with learning difficulties. We pay taxes for public service professionals to work with those enduring behavioral problems. We pay taxes to house individuals with mental retardation. We pay taxes to build more jails because many individuals with FAS or FAE unwittingly get in trouble with the law.

Also, what about the immeasurable costs like the guilt or low self-esteem of the mother of a FAS/FAE child? Or the emotional anguish of those connected to a child with behavioral problems? Or the inexplicable confusion and frustration of actually growing up with a learning difficulty? There are many hidden costs associated with these invisible, but preventable, challenges that FAS/FAE youngsters have to endure.

The myth that "only a couple of drinks won't hurt" is a dangerous one. And who is to judge the potency of a couple of drinks? To some, a couple of drinks may be two shots of straight rum on the rocks. To others, four glasses of champagne is nothing. Is it a tumbler or a shot, a small or a large glass? How do you measure the limit? What is even considered the limit? To most professionals working with pregnant mothers, there still remains a mystery as to when too much alcohol becomes too much. We adults may tolerate a variable amount. An unborn child may tolerate very little. Nobody really knows. Because of this mystery, even a couple of glasses of wine each day may jeopardize the well-being of an unborn child. And refraining from drinking alcohol only during the first three months is still questionable. Remember, the fetus is developing for the entire nine months of pregnancy, not just in the first trimester.

How can those who are not pregnant help those who are? By exercising some compassion. Realize that it can be a gift to support a pregnant mother by enclosing her into the folds of any celebration, any party, any good moment—without the alcohol. In so doing, we are not denying alcohol, but just having a good time without the alcohol. So help, by eliminating any temptation. After all, being pregnant is only for a small period of time in one's life.

Louise Erdrich writes in the foreword of her husband's book, *The Broken Cord* (by Michael Dorris, Harper & Row, 1989), a story about their adopted son born with FAS, the following.

> . . . go and sit beside the alcohol-affected while
> they try to learn how to add. My mother, Rita
> Erdrich, who works with disabled children at
> the Wahpeton Indian School, does this every
> day. Dry their frustrated tears. Fight for them in
> the society they don't understand. Tell them
> every simple thing they must know for survival,
> one million, two million, three million times.
> Hold their heads when they have unnecessary

seizures and wipe the blood from their bitten
lips. Force them to take medicine. Keep the
damaged of the earth safe. Love them. Watch
them grow up to sink into the easy mud of
alcoholism. Suffer a crime they won't understand committing. Try to understand their lack
of remorse. As taxpayers, you are already paying
for their jail terms, and footing the bills for
expensive treatment and education. Be a victim
yourself, beat your head against a world of brick,
fail constantly.

Of *The Broken Cord*, the *Detroit News* said, "The deeply moving and fierce story of Michael Dorris' search for answers.
Part memoir, part mystery, part love story, polemic and social
and public health story, this is the rare book that focuses attention like a magnifying glass on a hot sunny day. It burns."
The *New York Times Book Review* had this to say, "*The Broken
Cord* should be required reading for all medical professionals
and social workers, and especially for pregnant women, and
women who contemplate pregnancy, who may be tempted to
drink." Also, it should be required reading for all politicians,
purse holders who grant money for prevention of FAS/FAE
and educational pregnancy programs, plus required reading
for any of us who might put a glass of alcohol into a pregnant
woman's hand. Think about it. We are all responsible for raising healthy children, not just the mother. After all, once born,
these children become the newest members of our society—
of our collective society in which we are all members.

What else? In "Taking Charge," author Irene Pollin dis-
cusses the benefits of support groups in an issue of the
National Organization on Fetal Alcohol Syndrome Newsletter.
She writes: "You can say *nothing*, and you're going to get answers to a lot of your questions hearing other people's stories.
Suddenly you're finding a way. So, really, the dynamic of the
whole process that's going on is extremely helpful, especially
if it's run by a good professional."

Learning Disorders

For some people—from Albert Einstein to Whoopi Goldberg, Magic Johnson to Cher—going to school was a trying experience. They all had, or have, a learning disability. This is no surprise. Learning disabilities (LD—which also stands for "Lotsa Determination") have been around a long time. It goes back for centuries.

Today, according to the National Center for Learning Disabilities (NCLD), between ten and fifteen percent of the American population is learning-disabled. Often, LD runs in families. And it never goes away. Actually, because this is a "hidden handicap" and difficult to diagnose, the figure of those affected is probably higher. Believed to be neurological in origin, LD comes in many forms. LD primarily involves a mix-up in the way information is stored, processed or produced in the brain. Its origin has nothing do with behavioral problems, though it can result in behavioral difficulties. These problems often are overlooked or misunderstood, and individuals, primarily children, with LD find their self-esteem suffering, suffering a great deal. Adequate diagnostic, educational or training services are often unavailable. Because of this, many never reach their full potential, and can become a school dropout, a delinquent, or a substance abuser, to name a few horrors.

It's frustrating because many people with LD have average to above-average intelligence. LD affects one's ability to read, write, speak, or compute math. It does not, however, affect intelligence. Einstein can be an example here, as his LD made simple arithmetic difficult for him to do; but the LD obviously had little impact on his intelligence. But not being able to read or write well can have serious consequences. One example of this is that persons with LD can be considered mentally retarded, never receive proper treatment, and sometimes can even end up being institutionalized. Horrible. So the need is to create awareness, provide early diagnoses, and follow up with appropriate intervention.

According to NCLD, some common characteristics of LD include problems with:

- Reading, writing, speech, and math

- Perception of time and space

- Concentration and attention

- Short-term memory

- Fine motor coordination

- Organization

- Self-esteem

- Socialization

While a learning disability cannot be outgrown, its effect can be lessened and compensated for with proper attention and treatment. "Students with LD can be helped dramatically by computer technology" says Barbara S. Heinisch, associate professor, Department of Special Education, and director of the Adaptive Technology Lab at the Southern Connecticut State University. Because of the computer's varied programs and ability to create solutions, Heinisch goes on to say, "One of the greatest benefits of computer use for students with LD is that they never have to see their written work in an inferior state . . . allowing them to produce work which is indicative of their true abilities." How indescribably liberating.

Dyslexia

One common form of LD is dyslexia, the problem of not being able to read accurately, despite the ability to see and recognize most letters. It's a condition involving poor visual processing and the way the brain interprets the visual message. Individuals with dyslexia can demonstrate a myriad of symptoms. This might include forgetting what has been read, poor comprehension or attention span, sloppy writing, doing work slowly, or expressing excessive frustration despite a healthy mental disposition. Fortunately, dyslexia is a largely treatable and livable condition once properly diagnosed. However, these individuals often are labeled "dyslexic." We should remember, it's a condition, not a person. Once this distinction is made and people respond to the condition instead of reacting to the person, self-esteem can flourish among persons with any kind of LD.

Unfortunately, our educational system tends to handle learning disorders by seeking the best way to teach a "problem" child. This does not correct the disorder, but results in working around the problem. Fortunately, the medical model's aim is to identify and correct the core disorder. This is particularly important in vision because so much of what we learn depends upon a highly functioning visual system.

Chronic Fatigue Immune Dysfunction Syndrome

Take another not-so-visible condition: the chronic fatigue immune dysfunction syndrome (CFIDS), also referred to as the chronic Epstein-Barr virus or the yuppie flu. Though no one has precise figures, epidemiologists estimate that two to five million Americans have been stricken. And, as mentioned before, these estimates are always low for a variety of reasons.

It has been called "the disease of the nineties," yet it is probably not a new disease. Some believe that Florence Nightingale and Charles Darwin may have had it. Disabling? Researchers guess that a third of the people with CFIDS in this country today are nearly totally bedridden. Another third are disabled in that these people cannot hold jobs, let alone plan the next day's activities. The other third remain quite functional and employed with some major adjustment to their lifestyle and daily activity. Yet, most of these people look "normal" to us.

The medical profession still tends to believe that CFIDS is an attitude and not an illness. Many medical people have been treating it as a non-disease, as a product of stress, or as a psychosomatic problem. Why? Some thinking here, according to the National CFIDS Foundation, is that CFIDS affects twice as many women as men, and historically diseases primarily affecting women have not been treated seriously by the medical profession.

The Foundation further postulates that, as a society, we are slow to recognize growing epidemics and often discount them in their early stages due to fear—much as with the AIDS epidemic. Too, there is no easily accessible laboratory test to diagnose CFIDS. Yet, epidemiological evidence is mounting to the effect that this disease is very real and very serious, invisible as it may seem.

The Tip of the Iceberg

This initial discussion of invisible disabilities is merely the tip of the tip. The iceberg below runs deep. As always, there is more. Invisible as these disabilities may seem, visible consciousness and awareness are needed on all our behalf. Remember, very few of us are "normal." Remember something Elisabeth Kübler-Ross says, "I'm not okay, you are not okay, so that's okay." In so many ways, acknowledging and understanding that we are not, in many ways, perfect is a perfect way to be.

CHAPTER

4

INVISIBLE-TO-VISIBLE DISABILITIES

What may start out as an invisible disability can end up as a visible disability. A few obvious examples are arthritis, multiple sclerosis, diabetes, ALS. The process of going from an invisible disability to a visible disability usually signifies a worsening of the condition. However, the degree of visibility in no way indicates the degree of disability an individual may experience.

What these conditions—invisible or visible—do share in common is the absolute requirement of infinite coping skills. Dealing with the unknown means living an unpredictable life, mildly stated. It means an upheaval of any and all future plans. It means living in the very present, from day-to-day. It means a realigning of priorities. It means getting a Ph.D. in Copability.

In coping are revealed the pluses as well as minuses of the upheavals in our lives. The plus factors, such as the realigning of priorities, are strong and reassuring. Personally, my spirituality, and my growth in becoming more spiritual, have become very important. (I share some of this with you in the

51

last chapter.) Too, realizing just how vulnerable I was made me quite cognizant of how fragile life can be. The hidden benefit? There is more open love in my life. In other words, I've got nothing to lose, so I give it all—and get so much in return. I may have very little material stuff in my name, but if you ask me, I feel inconceivably rich in life.

In fact, as I was working on this very chapter, a friend wrote to me, "I am in awe of your generous nature and the nature of your pure Spirit." And I responded, "There is nothing to be in awe about. You have it, too. It's just a matter of feeling it within, sharing the entire gamut, and pulling it out of others. That's all. No big deal."

Interestingly, the current thinking about the link between disability and religion is positive. The paradigm is shifting once again. Instead of thinking of disability as the result of bad karma or as a punishment, having a disability means you have been touched by God/dess/Moses/Buddha/whatever— a belief that existed centuries ago in great civilizations such as Greece. In other words, it was felt that persons with a disability were carrying more than just a burden, they were carrying a message from God. And thus, the revered position a person with a disability held in ancient history—and per- haps—holds once again today, is something to think about.

Back now to more earthly matters, about coping with some of the initial changes in my life.

On Coping

Copability . . . I first coined that word back in 1986 when I began getting slowed down by multiple sclerosis. Living in the country at the time, and loving every minute of rural ac- tivities, I wrote a letter to the *Mother Earth News* magazine *(TMEN)* asking its readers for suggestions and insights as to how others managed to cope while losing their mobility. The letter was published in the March-April 1987 issue of *TMEN*. Response was, true to *TMEN* readership, tremendous. And lengthy, touching, and inspiring. Most asked about my health, circumstances, and how I was managing. Many pointers and ideas were suggested. Reference materials often accompanied the letters. My file became five inches thick. I was over-whelmed—mostly by the gentleness and love that everybody shared with me then.

Not everyone who responded had a disability. There were some who wrote because of name recognition. Some were physical therapists or otherwise working in the helping field. And others simply wanted to share a bit of inspiration. A number did write regarding their own personal experiences in dealing with a disability and carrying on with life. They had done so with back problems (six percent), arthritic con-ditions (twelve percent), multiple sclerosis (twenty-seven per-cent), bad asthma (twenty percent), loss of limb (thirteen percent), and twenty-two percent with unidentified conditions.

I pondered the possible responses to the onslaught of let-ters, my thoughts ranging from handwriting a personal letter to jumping into a camper van and traveling the country to visit all who wrote. It meant that much to me. Of course, all these brainstorms were mere fantasies. Like most people, I lived with the daily reality of work, watering and weeding, cooking, and sleeping. And not necessarily in that order. But they were priorities none the less. So I came up with the idea of a newsletter. A labor of love. A response. The title? *Copability.*

In the newsletter, I described my circumstances, my health, how I was coping, and then some. What I was experiencing emotionally at the time is the following:

> Fate and faith is an interesting dance, so I've discovered recently. I guess they follow each other in that order. Having been so slowed down these past few months has been like riding a river raft: I'm over stiller waters now, but deeper too. I have had a chance to dive off, to deep crawl, to sense both the depth and the strength of the current. Riding ripples, as I did a lot of in the past, is too fast, and of course, too shallow. Swimming the deeper waters takes a bit of courage, strength, and oxy-gen. With the lack of coordination that has occurred,

there has been the added grace of understanding and love. I thought I had that already, but as a friend once said, "Nobody can predict a surprise!" I have seen something new—how kind people really are. Walking with a cane, slowly, causes people to rush to the door and hold it open for me. They look into my eyes. And smile. Now this is very new. I've usually done this for others. The effect is that of a softening, not self-pity, of added renewal and faith in people, including myself. So the fate of getting slowed down to see this has certainly been the positive side. That does not mean there are frustration-free days. Like all mortals, I feel the vulnerability walking right alongside me. I get scared or overwhelmed or simply tired. Also, I am aware that at such moments, I have to do one of two things immediately: either be with another human being or go into the garden, preferably both. As soon as I am with someone else, the focus is on this person. I pull out of myself that way. I feel their aches, their sharingness, their goodness, whatever. And of course, the garden is a place that consistently reeks of resurgence, of life, of response to my efforts. A nice rescue, always.

Since then, my ability to cope, also known as copability, had grown not so much larger, but deeper. I had found fibers of strength unbeknownst to me. Along this line of thought, I share with you a letter I received from one *TMEN* reader:

> Life is a wonderful thing and we constantly have to make changes. Some are easy to accept and others we can't even begin to understand why.

> However, here is my tip. Take one day at a time and learn how to enjoy what you can do. Even so small. Write it down. After a while the list grows long. If you get tired, rest, take deep breaths, and look around you. You will find something to appreciate. I once knew a man who built a stone wall one small stone at a time. The wall lives on for all to admire and wonder

who built such a wall. He took pride in what he
did one stone at a time. The wall had many
open places for people to come and go. We all
must come and go, and as we do, reach over the
wall even in a small way and help another
through the open places.

I have back nerve damage. It has turned my life
upside down. Age thirty-four, married with
three children under six years of age. Good luck.
Yours truly, DP, Lebanon, MO.

And I continued:

I struggle, no 'bout adoubt it, as we say in this neck of
the woods. Fatigue is as steady and close as my shadow,
so I make sure it doesn't get too long by working on my
Ph.D. in catnapping. I concentrate on Dr. Swank's low-
fat diet and miss the butter from time to time. I ma-
neuver the frustrations, like sitting on the ground while
digging a hole, instead of falling. I avoid emotional stress
by nipping things at the bud instead of allowing build-
ups. And I let myself laugh deeper these days. In essence, I follow Dr. Norman Vincent Peale's recipe. It is
a good one:

You've got a life to live. It's short, at best. It's a
wonderful privilege and a terrific opportunity—
and you've been equipped for it. Use your
equipment. Give it all you've got. Love your
neighbor—he's having just as much trouble as
you are . . .

Multiple Sclerosis

Many people ask about my disability, multiple sclerosis (MS).
Equally, a number of people confuse MS with muscular dystrophy (MD). They are two very different conditions. MS
affects the nerves and MD affects the muscles. Actually, MS
has a lot more in common with other chronic illnesses such
as the Epstein-Barr virus (chronic fatigue immune deficiency

syndrome), systemic lupus, and environmental illnesses. A major factor that all share is unpredictability. Our conditions vary from day to day, week to week, year to year. This unpredictability is most chronic.

MS is a neurological disorder that is the result of an autoimmune attack on the nerve sheath, also known as the myelin sheath. As a result of these attacks, the myelin sheath, an insulation that surrounds message-carrying nerves, gets stripped. Consequently, messages coming from the brain never make it to their final destinations. They short out in the exposed areas that have been stripped of myelin. What we then experience can be weakness, tingling, numbness or other impaired sensations, poor coordination and balance, poor eyesight, slurred speech, spasticity or stiffness of muscles, tremors, sensitivity to heat, and a host of other things.

A person who has MS usually experiences different combinations of these symptoms, sometimes in odd episodes and sometimes with progressive severity. It is predictably unpredictable for everyone. Some people have a very mild case. For others, the illness can result in reliance on a wheelchair and then some. For many, it involves a series of attacks, called exacerbations, followed by partial or complete recovery, known as remissive periods or remission. Others experience symptoms that remain stable over many years; and some experience symptoms that gradually worsen over time. But for all, it is predictably unpredictable.

There is no understanding of its cause. Theories abound. Some say it is a result of genetic disposition. Some theorize that it is environmental, since known clusters of the disease occur in certain areas throughout the country. Some say it is a virus.

At present, there is no cure. The loss of myelin cannot be reversed. Though the impact of this autoimmune disease can be modified through adjustments, adaptations, and some medications, it is a demanding and lifelong process to which we must respond. A phenomenal amount of patience and humor is required in dealing with a body that is predictably uncooperative. Also, the ability to pace oneself and to rest is paramount. I often refer to this as my "obtaining a Ph.D. in pacing." And as with many diseases, stress, emotional or physical, does not help. So learning how to successfully manage stress in one's life is equally crucial.

Because MS in itself is not a fatal disease, finding a cure is not as pressing as finding a cure for cancer or AIDS. Yet, MS is very debilitating and affects more than just the person who has it. Like any disabling condition, it impacts the surrounding people as well. For example, MS can be extraordinarily difficult for those who are parents. The ability to parent gradually subsides with the increasing onset of the disease. And it can wreck havoc on primary relationships. On the job, work can be more difficult on account of fatigue. Because it initially often shows up in persons between the ages of twenty and forty years, the so-called prime years, a certain vitality is undermined. Most people simply do not understand this. In fact, newly diagnosed individuals may have a hard time comprehending what they are experiencing, precisely because of all the unknowns, the unpredictability, and the reactions of those surrounding them. It is a most insidious condition.

Recently, an international conference held in Atlanta, Georgia, specifically addressed issues concerning MS. One topic included the question of who, as members of the media, do we need more to address concerning MS: the newly diagnosed or those who have been living with MS for a while? It is like asking, "What is preferable: to be born with a disability or to become disabled later on in life?" Though we may have our thoughts about the above, there are no easy answers.

Think about it. Being born with a disability means you are handling a doubled-edged sword. Starting with Day One, you are dealing with both the disability and how people relate to you. Chances are you will be pitied, will be treated differently, and will never experience true independence as most of the nondisabled world knows it. As part of your shadow, there will be a label unwittingly given to you by others. You'll see shapes in your shadow that bear no resemblance to the shape of the real you. A lousy deal, if you ask.

Then there are those of us who became disabled—read that as diagnosed with MS—later on in life. In the prime of our life, a boulder gets thrown in our creek, and its flow loses a familiar direction. The water backs up and stagnates. In this blockage, the water not only develops a muddy state—read that as unclear—but is phlegmatic, torpid, and very dull—just the kind of environment mosquitoes love. Oftentimes it is during this period that our relationships go awry. Our careers are jeopardized. Many of us cannot handle school anymore. Any way you look at it, the half-full cup becomes a can of worms. A lousy deal, if you ask.

But because of the forever-changing nature of MS, I feel that both the newly diagnosed and those who have lived with MS for a while need constant addressing, always, and in all ways. Too, we individuals who have lived with MS for a while owe it to comfort the newly diagnosed. Thus the constant need to stay further in touch.

For a long time, many of us lived in the fear of the unknown. And, for most of us, the diagnosis was usually slow in coming. Too, the initial stretch shortly after being diagnosed was indeed a frightening period. The local chapter of the National Multiple Sclerosis Society where I live knows this. One of the best and most well-received seminars the chapter gives has the old timers speak to the newly diagnosed. And what shared wisdom occurs at these gatherings—I wish such had existed when I was newly diagnosed myself. As panel members, we find ourselves conveying the message, "Yes, there is life after diagnosis."

In fact, though unaware of any other panel members' plan for their talks, we not only communicate similar messages, but also often refer to the same quotations. Each time, every speaker feels that having a good attitude is paramount, whether you are a newcomer or an old timer living with MS. Because our gears are constantly shifting, we need to do a good lube job, constantly greasing our gears with a positive attitude.

Diabetes

Everyone knows someone with diabetes. How true. Even yours truly just has to look out of her living room window at the neighbor across the street who lives with diabetes. It is that close. For many of us, it is also that prevalent.

Not only is my neighbor's life complicated by diabetes-related difficulties such as sores that are slow to heal, frequent gum infections, numbness in her feet — she lost her husband in 1994 (also a person with diabetes) to a probable diabetic-related stroke. In fact, it is common knowledge among health professionals that people with diabetes are five times more likely to suffer a stroke.

The American Diabetes Association (ADA) claims that over 14 million people in the United States have diabetes, yet more than half of these are not aware they have the disease. Also, it is the fourth-leading cause of death by disease in the United States. Whew.

Diabetes has no cure as yet. But it's manageable for some by taking insulin shots or oral medication, for many by losing weight, for all by exercising or a combination of the above.

Exactly what is diabetes? The ADA explains that it is a chronic disease in which the body does not produce or properly use insulin, a hormone that converts sugar, starches and other foods into the energy we need in our daily lives. There are two types of diabetes. Type I is called insulin independent, an autoimmune disease in which the body does not produce any insulin whatsoever. Most often children and young adults, people with Type I diabetes must take daily insulin injections to stay alive. Only 5 percent of those diagnosed with diabetes get this type. Type II, the non-insulin-dependent and more common form, is known primarily to be a metabolic disorder. Here, the body is not able to make enough insulin or properly use it. In essence, the body is deprived of absorbing the necessary fuel to remain healthy. As a result, we starve parts of our body. Then, these parts malfunction.

No one knows what causes diabetes, although genetics and obesity appear to play significant roles. Also, apparently, members of certain ethnic groups are at greater risk. Too, if you are over forty years and overweight, your risk increases. Interestingly, mothers with high-birth-weight babies — weighing more than nine pounds at birth — are also at risk.

Many folks only become aware of their diabetes when they develop one of its complications such as blindness, kidney disease, amputation, heart disease, or stroke. Diabetes is known to be the leading cause of adult-onset blindness. Each year, from 15 to 39 thousand people lose their sight between the ages of twenty-five and seventy-four because of diabetes. Ten percent of all people with diabetes develop kidney disease. According to the ADA, more than 13 thousand people started treatment in 1990 for end-stage renal disease (kidney failure). Diabetes is the most frequent cause of nontraumatic lower limb amputations. Again, the ADA says, "The risk of a leg or foot amputation is 27.7 times greater for a person with diabetes." These numbers tell a frightening story. The expenses represent 5.8 percent of personal health costs in the United States, yet diagnosed diabetes patients account for only 2.8 percent of the total population. And again, about 7 million folks out there do not know they even have diabetes.

Arthritis

The chances of your knowing someone who has some form of arthritis are equally pretty good. According to the statistics, about 41 million Americans are affected by this disease. That adds up to one in every seven people, or, if you are family-oriented, one in every three families. And the family members are to be counted as well, as they are certainly affected by the rippling impact arthritis can have. In short, we are talking about a lot of people who are affected, either directly or indirectly, by this ever so prevalent disease.

Arthritis is considered a serious disease and a chronic one, meaning it can last on and off throughout one's life. There are over a hundred kinds of arthritis, mostly affecting our joints. Some of the other more well-known forms of arthritis include rheumatoid arthritis, lupus, gout, bursitis, tendinitis, and fibrositis.

Known as one of the oldest and most common diseases, arthritis causes the breakdown of tissues, specifically the cartilage that allows our joints to move properly. Arthritis has been considered the result of the normal wear and tear of our joints over a lifetime. Most people over sixty have it to some degree, due to the buildup of joint damage from either injuries or mere usage and stress over time.

Although arthritis can occur in any joint, it usually affects only one or two joints and doesn't spread further. Most commonly, these are weight-bearing joints such as the hips, knees and feet as well as the spine. Oddly, arthritis is also seen in the joints closest to the fingertips, resulting in the fairly common presence of bony growths there.

Among all the different types of arthritis, pain is the common denominator. Pain is a constant, and looming, issue for those with this disease. According to the Arthritis Foundation, "Chronic pain can be the worst part of having arthritis." Consequently, it can be debilitating, both physically and psychologically. Pain resulting from arthritis tends to isolate people socially. As many of you have experienced, the last thing you want to do is visit others when you have a painful headache or toothache. Pain can get in the way of many things, and this places added pressure on the families — to do or not to do becomes a repeated question and concern for all. For the individual involved, it is stressful to be so torn between decisions — whether to cope with the pain and go out under such circumstances or to stay home and try to relax. Many times, one succumbs to staying home because it seems to be easier, thus becoming isolated. And isolation is a factor leading to depression. A vicious circle.

Amyotrophic Lateral Sclerosis (Lou Gehrig's Disease)

What do (or did) jazz musician Charlie Mingus, actor David Niven, photographer Eliot Porter, classical musician Dmitri

Shostakovich, and some members of the San Francisco 49ers have in common? Or to be more obvious, add physicist Stephen Hawking and baseball great Lou Gehrig to the list.

All have, or had, the disease amyotrophic lateral sclerosis (ALS). According to numerous sources, ALS is a progressive neuromuscular disease that currently affects 20 thousand Americans. There are about 5 thousand newly diagnosed cases per year or fourteen new cases per day here in America.

Why haven't you heard much about it? Well, sad to say, life expectancy after diagnosis is short, usually twenty-four to thirty-six months, five years on occasion, and very rarely, as with physicist Stephen Hawking, decades. Therefore, not as many individuals are alive with ALS at any one point in time. So with reason, it has been called the silent killer. Yet, if we look at the ALS incidence (the number of new cases diagnosed each year), we see that it approximates the well-known neurological disease, multiple sclerosis, and is actually greater than that of muscular dystrophy.

More commonly known as Lou Gehrig's disease, since it became well known when he was diagnosed with it in 1939, ALS has been medically recognized over a hundred years. In fact, it is now estimated that ALS is responsible for one out of every thousand deaths in people over twenty.

Described as "a front-row seat to your own demise" by one individual with ALS, this progressive neuromuscular disease usually strikes adults between the ages of thirty-five and sixty-five, men about twice as often as women.

It is a disease that attacks the nerve cells controlling the movement of our voluntary muscles. As a result, it causes the motor neurons to disintegrate and results in the wasting away, or atrophying, of muscles. Usually first to be affected are the legs and arms. And, of course, paralysis of these appendages follows. Eventually, the muscles responsible for speech, chewing, and swallowing atrophy. Then . . .

Kathleen J. Namors of Lisle, IL, whose brother was diagnosed at the age of thirty-eight, writes,

> Imagine not being able to control a single
> muscle or [not] being able to execute normal
> functions—no walking, no writing, no smiling,
> no talking, no eating, and then . . . no breathing.
> Yet, through this torment, the mind and the
> senses remain unaffected.

Whew. How horrifying. Did Jean-Paul Sartre have this in mind when he wrote the play, *No Exit?*

Barry H. Goldberg of Plano, TX, writes:

> I am beating the odds because, as I write this,
> I've had ALS for more than three years. I can
> best describe its impact by what I miss as the
> disease progresses . . . I simply miss walking. I
> used to miss playing the guitar; now I miss
> blowing my own nose, feeding myself and going
> to the bathroom myself . . . I used to miss my
> wife at work; now I miss the opportunity for her
> to work because she had to quit to care for me
> twenty-four hours a day. I used to miss holding
> my wife's hand; now I miss holding my wife.

There is a very poignant story related by Albuquerque's Helen Renwick, in her article, "To the Physician Who Cared Enough to Ask." It reveals her feelings about not being told, when obviously first displaying ALS symptoms in 1989, that she had Lou Gehrig's disease. Dictated to her friend and caretaker, Pat Simmons, six months before she died (February 24, 1995), Helen concludes:

> Yes, my physician friend, since there is no cure
> for ALS, it would behoove those in your profes-
> sion to change the way they do business with
> patients and families. The diagnosis was *not*
> [Helen's emphasis] the hard part. The *hard part*
> has been the fears of how I will survive in the
> interim between diagnosis and death. *What if*
> the focus of physicians had been to help me face
> what I had to face in the most open and com-
> passionate way possible?

Epilepsy

Though epilepsy is an invisible condition, it becomes visible when a seizure occurs. Epilepsy. The dictionary (*Webster's*, 2nd Ed.) says in part, *ep'i.lep'sy:* a seizure, the "falling sickness." It also has been called, the "hidden handicap." Until . . .

I had grown up in a shroud of silence about epilepsy, so I decided to learn more about this so-called hidden handicap. I talked at length to persons living with epilepsy, read medical texts, read numerous Epilepsy Foundation of America (EFA) booklets, and watched videos. As a friend once said, "Education is the cure for ignorance." With this, I became determined to clear up my ignorance. Because most of us know so little about epilepsy—the word used for a host of seizure disorders—and know of someone, directly or indirectly with epilepsy, it's time we learn more.

Historically, "epilepsy" was the whispered word of those having a seizure: it was devil's work—or God's touch—depending upon your upbringing and current beliefs. Regardless, "epilepsy" has been, and still is, a loaded word, unfairly so. Because of the prejudice and stigma(s) attached, it is a very lonely condition. Even the medical profession remains relatively naive. Epilepsy may warrant, at most, three pages in a medical textbook, despite its having been around for a while. Many believe that Julius Caesar may have had it. Add to the list Richard Burton and Elton John. In other words, it has been around, lots.

It is still around. According to the EFA, one percent of our population has this condition by the age of twenty. Each year, there are a 125 thousand new cases of epilepsy in the United States alone. Currently, there are over 2 million people in this country with some form of active epilepsy according to the EFA. That is 2 million *known* cases of epilepsy. What about all those forced into denial of their condition? One person living with epilepsy has found in talking to those with seizure disorders that only about half openly acknowledge their condition. At time of diagnosis, thirty percent will be under age eighteen. That breaks down to over one and a half per thousand in preschool children. The figure is possibly higher today. But improved medication and early intervention are actually dropping the number of cases among children. More good news is with proper treatment, many children can outgrow the condition between the ages of nine and nineteen.

According to the medical publication *Organic Psychiatry*, by William Lishman, causes can vary from birth injury, congenital malformations, traumatic brain injury, strokes, infections of the brain, brain tumors, drugs, or toxins such as lead or the chlorinated hydrocarbons found in insecticides. This same publication emphasizes that epilepsy is not a mental disorder, but has an organic cause such as those listed above. Even someone with multiple sclerosis can occasionally get a seizure disorder because of the scarring of their brain nerves caused by MS. Something as simple as a firecracker can precipitate a seizure in one of our war veterans that has suffered a traumatic brain injury while on duty and has incurred epilepsy as a result. And so the misunderstanding that epilepsy is an emotional illness occurs often in the minds of casual observers. But I reiterate, this is not the case. It is understood, however, that emotional disturbances, shock or surprise, interpersonal stresses, or tensions can frequently trigger a seizure.

Many individuals with epilepsy imply it's not the condition that troubles them, but the way society responds to their neurological disorder. Even professionals in the medical field have difficulty dealing with epilepsy. Our odd attitudes about individuals with any kind of seizure disorder are quite pervasive. Precisely because of this, many of those with epilepsy fear having a seizure in public.

Writer Jodi McBride of Miami, a person living with epilepsy as a result of a childhood illness, was inappropriately institutionalized because she was misdiagnosed. Of this, she writes,

> I tried to explain it all to others, this altered state of mind
> Just to discover no one listened while I really tried to find
> An explanation for this world I didn't know.

Another state of being, another world where I spent so
   much time alone.
Two selves—and how could I explain
This different life I suddenly lived somewhere inside my
   brain?

Louise Hagan, an Albuquerque mother of two and a registered nurse, says that every time she has a seizure in public,
she goes home and cries. Others with epilepsy avoid such
encounters by simply staying home and are very isolated as a
result. What an utter shame. The loss of any kind of control
is a no-no in our society. Consequently, we are not very forthcoming with understanding or compassion—just what people
with epilepsy need.

So what are the best actions to take if someone has a con-
vulsive seizure?

- Stay calm.

- Move away surrounding sharp objects.

- Loosen tight clothes.

- Inform onlookers.

- Do not put anything in the mouth—it is
  impossible to swallow the tongue.

- Do not restrain the individual having a seizure.

If seizures last more than five minutes, if the individual is
injured, or if the individual is pregnant, call an ambulance.
After a seizure:

- Roll the person on their side.

- Observe and remember sequence of events.

- Be calm, supportive, and reassuring.

The most important thing is to let this person know after a
seizure what has happened and that everything is okay. Be
reassuring. Be compassionate. Participate in the Golden Rule:
give unto others what you would want to be given unto you.

CHAPTER 5

VISIBLE DISABILITIES

To discuss all the visible disabilities would require a book or two in itself, so I'll just write about two, namely blindness and mobility impairment.

On Blindness

According to a director of Newsline for the Blind, "Blindness is not what you think it is." Though not blind himself, he did spend two months as a blind person training at the Orientation Center in Alamagordo run by the New Mexico Commission for the Blind. Learning the tricks of the trade, so to speak, he came away from the training with a heightened acuity of his senses, with an awareness of other peoples' ignorance, and with an understanding that a blind person can just about do anything one wishes to do, short of driving a car.

What stopped him more than anything, was the attitude of others, their pity, and their interference with his doing things on his own. People grabbed his arm unexpectedly. People assumed he needed help. And people automatically equated his apparent blindness with poverty. He felt much of what Patricia Logan, a National Federation of the Blind member of the New York chapter, said in a letter to the media,

> I reject and condemn the inference and remarks
> which suggest that life without sight necessarily
> has to be one of almost total dependence on
> loved ones; a life permeated with depression and
> dominated by thoughts of what had been lost,
> rather than by the wealth of experiences based
> on what has been retained.

We can learn much here. Blind people exercise all their other senses a great deal, and in doing so, develop strengths in such areas, just as Arnold Schwarzenegger did in building his muscles. Blind people do not have ultra-hearing, but simply, are better listeners. To wit, by eliminating visual distractions at a musical concert with our eyes closed, we hear better. Added sensitivity as to where the sun rays are, when walking outdoors, can assist in orientation. This same sensitivity indicates a change in air pressure, a possible wall nearby, or a door opening up ahead.

Not all blind people are totally without sight. Once again, variations abound. There are those who have a sensitivity to light and dark. Some lack direct vision, but can see peripherally. Some were born blind, while others lost their sight later on in their lives. Many—and this is true to a certain extent for most all of our aging population—have difficulty reading small print, including yours truly. Awareness of these variations can help in our understanding of how someone might deal with their individual circumstances.

At this juncture, you are probably asking yourself, how can I best be in the company of a blind person?

• Be yourself, nothing more, nothing less.

• Let your voice indicate where you are. Touch
  only to shake hands.

• Do not offer help without first asking if you can
  be of assistance in any way. If the answer is no,
  relax. And enjoy one another.

- Guide dogs are on the job, not to be petted or crooned over. Leave them alone.

- Be honest. If you don't know to what extent blindness affects this individual, ask for clarity. After all, this individual is the expert, not you.

- Don't worry about using such words as "see." Even a blind person will say, "See you later."

About the thoughtless bias that blind individuals encounter, I have a story to tell. Most of us like animals. We people can be big, small, pregnant, Polynesian, deaf, blind, or a wheelchair user. Regardless, animals don't care—that is one thing these critters have over us: no thought of bias. And when we go to the zoo, we often have children in tow, in strollers, or even in wheelchairs, some of which are power chairs. In fact, when I go to the zoo, I go in my motorized rickshaw (a three-wheel scooter). The animals don't seem to mind. And when I go to the zoo, there are virtually always as many children as animals. So I watch both. The animals, meanwhile, probably are watching us. This business has been going on for years, worldwide. When something new crops up, naturally we're all curious, animals included. When someone's guide dog appears, of course the caged critters will be curious. Some zoo animals will react defensively, some will sniff, and some will be as nonchalant as ever.

As a result of a recent event here where I live, and the ensuing publicity, a couple of blind people with their accompanying guide dogs created some consternation at the local zoo. The ADA (Americans with Disability Act) allows the right for blind people to visit the zoo. But, according to the zoo keepers and the media, a recent visit of individuals who happened to be blind, and their accompanying guide dogs, turned into a test of animal versus animal. The keepers questioned whether guide dogs should even be allowed on the zoo grounds. The publicity also made others wonder, "Why would someone who can't see even want to go to the zoo?"

Granted, guide dogs may be a new phenomenon for the zoo animals, but at one time, so were power chairs. And so were children throwing not-so-quiet tantrums. Look at it this way: there is always a beginning to the new. The animals at our zoo don't seem to care much about the noises of screaming children or motorized rickshaws now. Of the aforementioned shrieking child, power chair, and guide dog, the guide dog seems to be the quietest. It goes without saying that by nature of their training and work, these dogs are extremely obedient, gentle, and aware. Think about it. Have you ever heard one bark? I haven't. Initially, the zoo animals may be curious or wary of the appearance of guide dogs. After all, this is a new sight for them. However, over time and with due familiarity, the zoo animals probably would not care about someone's guide dog. Any possible threat to the caged critters would become nonexistent. Like our knowing that most tigers come with stripes, the zoo animals would learn that some people come with dogs. Period.

Losing sight at the age of forty-two, Christine simply has never lost sight of her love for animals. In fact, taking her grandchildren to the zoo is, and has been, a great pleasure for Christine. And needless to say, family outings to the zoo are fun. But, for a long time, Christine did not go. Why? She did not want to have a confrontation in front of the kids with the zoo keepers about taking her guide dog. What a car is to a person, a guide dog is to a blind person: independence, freedom of movement, freedom of pace. Christine does not like hanging on to someone's elbow, just as we don't like riding the Greyhound bus while touring Yellowstone National Park—thus, we use our own car. This is like someone having his or her own guide dog for maximum freedom.

When at the zoo, Christine sees everything with her other senses and then some. She says,

> We all see in our own ways. We hear the
> children's expressions of delight. We smell
> everything. We feel the hot sun on the nape of
> our neck, the shade's cool spaces, and the

breezes ruffling our hair. I love the outdoors and
I love sharing all with my family. When we are
with the giraffes, I know what they look like
because I still have the visual memory from the
days before becoming blind.

Christine also emphasizes that her senses of hearing, smell-
ing, or feeling are not superior to anyone else's. She states
that now they are simply more sensitive from greater use. How
true. I did not become a better writer because my speech has
deteriorated with my condition. Simply, the writing has improved, and still improves, with practice and constant doing.
It's like playing the piano. Practice, practice, and you will play
with much greater acumen, fine tuning always. Too, Christine learns much about the person who may be describing the
scene for her. She says, "We all see with the mind's eye. From
five different people come five different interpretations of the
color red." What a gold mine of awareness.

Sadly, with today's rise in hate crimes, and within the disability community, blind individuals seem to be targeted a
great deal. Ironically, it is precisely because their disability is
so visible while the perpetrator remains so invisible. What
can we do? Since attacks occur randomly, you never know
when you will see one. And if you have witnessed such,
remain to be a witness, an ally.

Mobility Challenges

Between the following stories, and my letter to Jeffrey in
Chapter 2, the descriptions of some mobility challenges will
give you an inkling as to what they are and what they are not.

Though not always that apparent and not always affectng
mobility, the loss of a leg, foot, arm or hand due to accident is
more common than being born minus one of these appendages. Because of modern technology and medicine, a well-
fitted leg prosthesis and a pair of Levi's can make this particular
mobility challenge a little less obvious.

Not surprisingly, in a United Nations (UN) meeting on the International Day of Disabled Persons held in December, 1995, Mamadou Barry, chief of the Disabled Person Unit, reported one of the greatest, current causes of disability: land mines. As I write this, it is estimated by the State Department that nearly 2 thousand people, worldwide, are killed or injured by land mines each month (ninety percent of the victims are civilians). There are still approximately 100 million live mines in over sixty-five countries.

Most of these mines are in third world countries. A loss of an appendage is the most common injury survivors endure. Most of these countries do not have the medical technology, nor the finances, that would enable them to provide decent prostheses to allow the survivors a greater freedom of movement or any kind of independence.

Many of us have seen the bumper sticker, "Practice random kindness and senseless acts of beauty." But how many of us have followed this advice more than once this year? Is it something you do only around the holiday season or truly spontaneous, timeless acts of kindness or beauty? About this, let me tell you a story.

One act of beauty was done by a University of New Mexico student of Ecuadorian heritage, Manuel Garcia. A couple of years ago he went to Ecuador to visit relatives. He learned for the first time that his cousin, Marcos, had outgrown a series of badly made artificial leg prostheses for his right leg, amputated as a result of an childhood accident. Manuel, who at the time lived in Iowa, returned home rather concerned. He talked to doctors at the Iowa Medical Clinic in his hometown, to members of his church, and to people in the surrounding community, all of whom ended up sponsoring Marcos' trip up to Iowa for a new, properly-fitted prosthesis.

As Marcos said, "In my country, it is difficult to make a prosthesis in a good way." The ones made in Ecuador never fit him very well, often leaving sores and blisters on his stump as he grew up. So he arrived in Iowa using crutches, and was properly fitted with a new, well-made prosthesis. He left walking on his own. The act of beauty? For the first time ever, the then twenty-seven-year-old Marcos could carry his two-year-old son.

On a trip to Central America, Ralf Hotchkiss of Berkeley, California, found wheelchairs a rare sight there. The few available ones were imports, very expensive, and old tanks at best. In a random act, Hotchkiss pieced one together out of materials existing down there. He understood its value, being a wheelchair user himself. Like Manuel, he returned home concerned. And continued to fiddle with the idea of building cheap wheelchairs. Today, as a result, detailed and descriptive literature goes out to countries where people are in dire need of wheelchairs. He designs wheelchairs utilizing available, on-site materials. His is an act that allows many to see the sunrise for the first time.

Because others describe life in a wheelchair so well, I recommend other readings. To begin, I highly recommend the novel, *The Body's Memory,* by Jean Stewart (St. Martin's House, 1993). The novel is largely based on Stewart's own experiences. With a degree in botany, she worked one and a half years in agrochemical research at a large pharmaceutical firm. Part of her job was testing toxic herbicides. Out of personal ethics, she quit when discovering the firm had Defense Department contacts. Six years later, doctors found a tumor in her hip muscle, one of the body's most common reactions to dioxin ("Agent Orange") herbicide exposure. Today, Stewart is a disability activist largely known by her writings and community actions. With profound accuracy, sensitivity, and passion, Stewart writes about what someone experiences and feels about becoming disabled later in life.

In a very readable fashion, Stewart's novel also provides penetrating insight of current disability issues. You do not, however, feel any didacticism or rhetoric concerning these issues. Instead, you are caught up with the novel's protagonist, Kate, and her story, her experiences, her rite of passage. In reading this book, the message of disablement is absorbed by osmosis. Stewart makes deft use of writers' techniques in describing both its central character, Kate, and her world of disablement. Because the story is so engrossing, and so beautifully written, you wish it would never end. Author Jean Stewart is another Annie Dillard. Although Stewart doesn't write about nature, she writes about disablement quite naturally in this first novel of hers. And Stewart writes well. It is an excellent read.

As an apropos follow-up to Stewart's novel, another book to rant and rave about is *Moving Violations: A Memoir* by John Hockenberry (Hyperion, 1995). As author Bill McKibben says about Hockenberry's book, "The world will seem different to you once you've read it, and there is no higher compliment for a book." Disabled or not, undoubtedly you equally will find it an excellent read. According to John Hockenberry, he wrote the story about being an award-winning television correspondent, National Public Radio commentator, political analyst, and journalist for several reasons. One reason was to tell what it is like to be different. His descriptions of life at waist-level are achingly honest, very funny, astute, and relentless.

There are many poignant moments in this book. In recounting one, Hockenberry tells of marrying his job supervisor. Though not a wheelchair user herself, she and John loved to roll downhill together. He describes the pursuit,

> Sitting on my lap . . . we were four arms, four
> legs, four wheels, one lap, two smiles, connected
> without rationalization. The wind cleansed our
> faces. The ride down the hill required no
> explanation. The wheelchair was a toy in free
> fall, the derby needed no soapbox. We were
> doing what anyone would have done with some
> wheels on a hill.

6

CHRONIC ILLNESSES
AND DISABILITIES

Another challenge to acknowledge is the difficult combination of a chronic illness and a physical disability. Did you ever think about dealing simultaneously with both a physical disability and a chronic illness? I never gave it a thought. Yet ironically, I have been living this very quandary. Multiple sclerosis is considered a chronic illness. In my case the result of this illness has been the paralysis of my legs, and more.

Chronic illness and permanent disablement happen to a lot of us. Tough. It's very tough. Usually, the chronic illness precedes the disabling condition, as with rheumatoid arthritis, multiple sclerosis, diabetes, or AIDS. Sometimes, it's the other way around, as with having polio first and later dealing with the post-polio syndrome. Regardless of order, the combination is difficult.

As I've mentioned, I have multiple sclerosis. So does Annette Funicello, and a host of others—like a friend of yours, a relative, a partner, a coworker—in short, more than a third of a million in this nation. Those of us facing, at the same time, a very unpredictable disease and a physical capability

75

that waxes and wanes, find any future planning equally erratic. But the above challenges seem mild when you consider the situation of a women of color who is disabled while also trying to cope with an ongoing illness. Too, she deals with the added hardships of being a woman and a person of color as well.

One of the hardest things about any of the aforementioned combinations, I think, is the unpredictability. It is tricky. You can't plan a dinner date a week down the road because you don't know how you will feel at the time or if the place, including the bathroom, will be accessible. As Bernie Siegel, M.D., reminds us, the most frequent question asked worldwide is, "Where is the bathroom?" Laughter aside, those of us who are facing such challenges find that life is not governed by a calendar, but instead is regulated by the physical accessibility of a place, and also by one's own unpredictable energy level.

I feel tremendously busy these days. I am. Though I could point to a myriad of reasons, the reality is that it takes more time to do anything, from getting dressed to getting in and out of the car. And much time is devoted to my well-being, making sure decent exercise, good eating, and rest occur on a daily basis. It makes for a busy day. After accomplishing the above, persons with a disability and a chronic illness then can relate to the family, go to work, to school, to see a play, visit with friends, have a light moment, and carry on with life. In every which way, we try to cope—endlessly. As the saying goes, "When the wind of changes blows, some build a shelter, others windmills." Unfortunately, the wind never stops blowing in this case.

As P.C. Andre says in the *MS Autobiography Book*, "This [his story] is not a story of heroics with sounds of drums and bugles and brightly colored banners flying. It is a story of choices." In essence, the choosing means prioritizing what you must or possibly can do that day. It means choosing to adjust to your mode of living—fighting, giving in or making the best of it. One's lifestyle constantly changes, much like the wind. Any prediction is definitely not part of our dialogue.

Talking about unpredictability, I wish the book, *Taking Charge: Overcoming the Challenges of Long-Term Illness*, by Irene Pollin with Susan K. Golant (Times Books, 1994) had been in print when I was newly diagnosed, for both myself and my family. It's certainly more than a how-to book. Because of Irene Pollin's own experiences, this book is like one of Sierra Club's trail guidebooks: well construed by an expert who has been there, more than once. I find so much accuracy and in-depth knowledge here that I take the liberty to quote Ms. Pollin a great deal in sharing this invaluable resource with you. She has much to share with us. Because Pollin comes from a place of measureless experience, she is a seasoned and well-qualified person to offer guidance to anyone of us dealing with a long-term condition, directly or indirectly.

Irene Pollin, M.S.W., lost both a son and a daughter to congenital heart disease. Of this, she says,

> As you can imagine, the loss of one child was extraordinarily painful. The loss of two, almost unimaginable. I sought counseling after my daughter [Linda] died and saw several well-trained professionals. Some prescribed tranquilizers, which served only to mask my feelings, not resolve them. Other therapists, rather than recognizing my children's illnesses and deaths as the source of my unhappiness, questioned me about my childhood.
>
> What I needed (and wasn't getting) from these counselors was coping with the long-term effects of heart disease on me and my family. It was then I realized that the mental health professionals receive little training specifically designed for those dealing with chronic illnesses. Few therapists are attuned to their *special needs* [author's emphasis].

Consequently she founded, and is currently president of, the Linda Pollin Foundation, " . . . which, with Children's Hospital in Boston (affiliated with Harvard University) supports the training of mental health professionals in their attention to the social and emotional needs of chronically ill patients." Once a year, in conjunction with the National Institute of Mental Health, the Pollin Foundation conducts a conference for physicians, psychiatrists, psychologists, and other health professionals around the country "to implement and support medical crisis counseling in hospitals and private practice settings nationwide."

Pollin refers to the "medical crisis counseling" because "I wanted the focus to be on the *medical crisis* [again the author's emphasis], not on personal or family history. During medical crisis counseling, I help my patients explore how their illness has affected their lives as well as those of their families. The medical crisis is the catalyst for their seeking help. The counseling is focused and short term . . . "

In this book, you are told what to expect, the upcoming challenges, and how best to deal with a chronic illness. But, Pollin says, "In reading *Taking Charge,* your goal should not be to cure your illness (for that may be impossible), but rather to learn how to live with it." She emphasizes, "Coping is a process that occurs over time and not overnight."

But more than just coping with a long-term illness, many other issues are discussed over the course of twelve chapters. Dealing with effective doctor-patient partnerships, changing relationships of any sort, fears and mastering these fears, and making attainable goals also are examined. The essence of *Taking Charge* is in addressing these fears. Pollin has found, as a result of both her experience and work, there are eight distinct fears that most with a long-term illness face. She confronts each fear in depth. They are:

- The fear of loss of control.

- The fear of loss of self-image.

- The fear of dependency.

- The fear of stigma.

- The fear of abandonment.

- The fear of expressing anger.

- The fear of isolation.

- The fear of death.

In addition, Pollin emphasizes that the wide range of powerful and painful emotions you and your loved ones may experience after a recent diagnosis of a long-term illness is to be expected and is perfectly normal.

But Pollin, fortunately, does not stop here. She takes things a step further by dealing with the reality of our situations and by recognizing helpful and attainable goals. Such aims include identifying our coping styles, decreasing anxiety and stress, improving cooperation with our doctors and nurses by understanding the framework from which they operate, and maximizing personal and environmental resources like physical strength, psychological stamina, support networks and knowledge.

And there is more. Pollin's epilogue is called "A Message of Hope." Hope is certainly the message here. Among all, I personally found the following as heartfelt, hopeful messages.

> "If you find ways to be valuable to your family
> and the community, you will never become a
> burden."

> "Society will not reject you unless you reject
> yourself."

> "You can attain a new (and satisfying) identity,
> but first you must let go of the old one."

There are not many books quite as enormously helpful as *Taking Charge*. Through Pollin's own personal and professional experience, she writes with unerring accuracy of what we experience and need. As a writer, prolific reader, disability advocate, and one who is living with a disabling chronic illness, I find *Taking Charge* a treasure.

It is a relief to find available this hand-holding guidebook. There are too many so-called how-to books out there that don't quite cut the mustard — or butter, if that is your preference — simply because the author(s), unlike Irene Pollin, lack a bona fide background, the experiential base that I consider a requirement for this kind of counseling.

We often find ourselves reading these helpful books to guide us through the physical and emotional territory of the unknown. There is nothing like a helping hand to hold on to while traveling unknown territory. In this case, we can count on Irene's hand. It is there.

PART TWO

Some Practical Matters

CHAPTER

7

CHILDREN AND
DISABILITIES

Due to a series of freak accidents, Beryl lost her right arm at the elbow and both legs at her hips. By the time I met her, she was traveling full-time throughout the Canadian provinces to teach children at schools about the world of disability. Beryl recounted a number of stories to me, including one of her more poignant moments. In this instance, she would call up a student, ask that child to grab a hold of "Stumpie," her amputated right arm, then ask that student to turn around and wave to watching classmates. She would say, "See, your hand is still there. It didn't fall off like your mom said it would if you touched me. Though not all of my parts are here, I am not contagious. I am simply an ordinary human being, like you. I am just short an arm."

There is nothing like a parent instilling fear into a naturally curious child. I have seen parents whisk the child away when asked why that lady is using the funny chair instead of walking. For children, such actions convey the impression that persons with disabilities are associated with something bad. Are these the values we want to give our young ones?

To reiterate the oft-said axiom, "Disability is a club any-one can join," is to repeat the truth over and over again. Dis-ability knows no bias. Poof—and you, your sister, your significant other, your dad, or anyone can unexpectedly end up using a cane or a wheelchair. How will your very own child react to *that?* Numerous parents have asked me, "What do you say under such circumstances? How do you teach young folks about disabilities?"

Children are naturally curious, and with such a state of mind, they are wonderfully open. Too, children smell untruth-ful responses the way a bear does dead fish, and children ac-cept straight-arrow replies as bears do honey. It is that natural. So teaching them, fortunately, is easier than it initially ap-pears. Beryl's example of contagion, or the lack of, is a great hit, and you bet it sticks with them for life.

Children come up to me all the time and ask why I use my wheelchair. I tell them my legs are no longer working and this chair serves as my legs now. You know what? They accept my chair as if it were their friend's bike. However, I do not tell the younger ones that my legs stopped working because of an illness, simply because I do not want children to fear that illness will make their legs stop working, a logical thought on their part.

This brings up another delicate point. Associations. I feel it is unwise to associate a disability with behavior, as some religions do. You know: the you-have-sinned-and-therefore-are-being-punished syndrome. As a possible result, children may become utterly fearful of their innocent mistakes, that God will get angry and that their legs will stop working as a result.

With the older ones, questions do persist. About myself, I answer them honestly, straightforwardly. I asked my four-teen-year-old friend, Brian, what he and his buddies would like to know about various disabilities. He replied, "Facts, like what is the cause and how does the person manage." Brian has watched me transfer, drive the car, do errands. And then, lose the ability to do so as I got worse. So he is fully aware of my disability, and so what? We still relate to one another, honestly, and very fondly.

What about children who have peers with disabilities? In this case, the responsibility of teaching your able-bodied child to understand the peer with a disability primarily falls on you. For example, your child has a classmate with cerebral palsy (CP). You are asked, "What is CP?" You don't know. The nicest thing you can do for your child is say, "I honestly don't know, but let's explore CP. Let's do this the way we do other projects. It is interesting and fun when we both learn together." And you call United Way for starts.

The key is teaching nonjudgmental facts. Facts, not myths. Remember, CP is a condition. It is not the result of a certain behavior. The classmate may be disabled, but not unable. Crutches may be needed to walk around, but actually, we are all in need of something, at some time. Grandma? She probably uses a walker now. The fact is her legs are tired from many years of use, and so she uses this tool to carry on. Likewise, I use wheels as a tool to get around.

Take Daddy. He may use glasses to see things more clearly. Take anyone, anything. You are not talking about something uncommon. Also you are teaching that disability is not synonymous with inability. People still manage with the help of their tools. You explain that we all have different needs and all have different tools. Teaching so, straightforwardly and honestly, is an action of love on your part, a step toward a more human approach. You are helping your child develop understanding, awareness, and acceptance. As a result, the classmate with a disability suffers less teasing and experiences greater acceptance. As adults, these kids' understanding of people with disabilities is one of respect, and the world becomes a better place for all of us to live.

Take Muthu, a nine-year-old with spina bifida, and her parents. In Muthu's short life, she has had a couple of major surgeries; is going to school; and is trying to work through her fears of India, having been so abused there before adoption. Over a very short period, I have watched Muthu blossom and grow well beyond her wheelchair in many ways. One of her parents was expressing the difficulties and frustration of getting Muthu a much needed decent, larger wheelchair. In despair and in talking about Muthu's life, her mom wished she could give more. Though a wheelchair may be slow in coming and though Muthu's legs may never allow her to run a marathon, she is getting from both parents the love, space, and permission to simply be. They may be small gifts, but they are gifts that will affect Muthu forever. Because of these gifts, Muthu's life undoubtedly will be one of quality, an ideal we all cherish. I am sure her parents realize this. The little things count—a great deal. Someone once said, "There is nothing really insignificant in this world and even great undertakings demand the honest, useful work of people who think they don't count."

Some parents have kids with disabilities. Some do not. But how many parents address their child's physical, emotional, and spiritual well-being at once? Everyone benefits by having such needs addressed, including the children with disabilities. The remark, "Children are like wet cement. Whatever falls on them makes an impression," says a great deal about influencing the ways children with disabilities can live their lives, now, and in the future.

Another story about Muthu. She is experiencing more difficult physical problems right now. But we can learn a great deal from her and her parents, in how they are all facing these challenges. The parents share with Muthu a mature and realistic appreciation of impermanence and vulnerability. Too, they instill pride in Muthu. As a result, Muthu does not have a hopeless attitude. She takes a delight in what life offers. She is feisty, intelligent, sensitive, and quite charming. From her parents, Muthu gathers strength to face her suffering. In fact, she recently said that "It is okay to die now—in my next life I probably will have legs that will work."

Now struggling to hold herself upright while playing the violin, playing wheelchair tennis, or simply playing with her friends, Muthu faces another major and risky surgery that involves fusing just about her entire spinal cord. But her parents finally said, "Enough." Muthu's parents have decided to journey back to India with her, despite the financial hard-ships, the wheelchair, and accompanying access obstacles. In doing so, they hope to continue meeting Muthu's physical, emotional, and spiritual needs. Muthu is going to the Dalai Lama's doctor in northern India for treatment instead of en-during an operation that has a questionable outcome and in-volves grave risks. She will be among Indian people, the people of her heritage. And she will experience further the spiritual depths her parents have already exposed her to through their Buddhist activities here in America.

What has been paralyzing Muthu is not only her condi-tion, but also the way society treats her. She is merely a physi-cal object to be "patched up" according to some doctors. She is another student "with problems" according to some people in the educational system. She is "just a pitiful kid in a wheel-chair who will be a burden for society in the future," thinks many a stranger. These inaccurate, painful beliefs run amok. I know. I have experienced this as well. Muthu and her parents have experienced it. And so have millions of others with dis-abilities. The disabled young, in particular, clearly are not given a chance with such ubiquitous attitudes.

At this point, you may pity Muthu's life. That is the far-thest thing she needs right now. Through all her trials and tribulations, she has gotten physical, emotional, and spiritual support from her parents. What gifts. But it is a shame to be calling the response to such needs a "gift" when it should be the norm. We have much to learn from Muthu and her folks. It is time to treat children with disabilities as fully engaged human beings, to share, to support, and to understand, re-gardless. Children are our future. Providing access is just one thing. Understanding fears, suffering, differences, feistiness or aspirations is another thing. Developing the spiritual is sending out a life raft of meaning. Making the child whole, disabled or not, is the idea.

So what about the children born with disabilities? Theirs is a loss that is greatly perpetuated by society which tends to view these children as "something less." And often, they are pitied by adults. Because of such stigmatizing attitudes, these children grow up carrying unnecessary burdens. In a way, they're never given a chance. To ease the problem, it is up to all of us to respect and treat any child, with or without a disability, as a whole person. To see this young person as a person, not as a "disabled child," empowers. And as a result, self-esteem, one of the hardest qualities to develop, simply escalates. This all helps to alleviate any sense of loss they may have.

In education, in recreation, more and more children with disabilities are interfacing these days with children who do not have a disability. I cannot sufficiently underscore the importance of this integration. All kids, regardless of ability, who experience such inclusion will certainly realize an improved social fabric in their lives. "Different" and "separate" will not exist in their vocabulary. But "acceptance" and "compassion" will.

Speaking of children and disabilities, let me mention again the question of Jerry Lewis and "his" children with muscular dystrophy (MD). Our perceptions of children with disabilities are, and have been, largely shaped by this man who has brought much attention to their needs. So why would anyone want to protest the efforts of Jerry Lewis in his money-raising telethons for the Muscular Dystrophy Association, and in particular, for children with MD? Where do the disagreements lie? Isn't he doing a good deed?

Well, yes and no. On prime-time television and before millions of viewers, Mr. Lewis referred to "his kids" with MD as "half persons." When questioned about that claim, he responded, "They can't run down the hall, can they?" But the "half person" issue really goes beyond having MD. There are a lot of us who "cannot run down the hall," including an infant learning to walk or an elderly parent recovering from a hip operation. And what about the unlucky weekend skier who needs to hobble about on crutches for six plus weeks? Because we cannot run down the hall, does that make us a "half person?" ? ?

The moot point here is not the money Mr. Lewis brings to the Muscular Dystrophy Association (MDA), but the ways he portrays children living with any kind of disability. And many persons with disabilities across the country are outraged by Mr. Lewis' conveying that children with disabilities are to be pitied, helpless, and dependent. He has done this for years and still continues to do so. This incorrect image that Lewis perpetuates flies in the very face of the movement among persons with disabilities to live autonomous, independent lives of quality and dignity—a movement that is now very widespread in our country and in the world. In fact, children with disabilities are given only a half perspective of themselves on being handed such an inaccurate label. Consequently, there are a lot of protesters out there. In fact, a number of previous "Jerry's Kids" have raised cain about him.

There is a movement among the "Jerry's Kids" who are now adults and calling themselves "Jerry's Orphans (JO)." They are demanding that the MDA get rid of Jerry; they are fed up with his "condescending paternalism," and his carrying "the attitude that stresses that, no matter what one does, life is meaningless in a wheelchair." Mike Ervin and Cris Matthews, previously part of Jerry's Kids and now activists in the JO group, state,

> We have borne the brunt of Lewis's pity in our lives as we struggle to live outside of institutions, as we struggle to find employment, as we struggle to develop meaningful relationships . . . We will fight until we end the paternalism that gives someone like Jerry Lewis the arrogance to decide the condition of our lives and remand us to perpetual babyhood.

These protesters are not against giving money to the MDA, but are asking that the MDA get rid of Jerry Lewis. They advocate a divestment plan which is simple: continue to give, but just don't give money during the Telethon, that's all. Be aware of the damaging images Jerry Lewis creates for all persons with disabilities, especially children.

In fact, according to the Research & Training Center on Independent Living, their guidelines for the media advise,

"The words and images you use can create a straightforward, positive view of people [read that as children] with disabilities or an insensitive portrayal that reinforces common myths and is a form of discrimination." At stake are issues involving children's dignity and rights. Children with disabilities are not to be pitied nor are they totally helpless and dependent. In their individual ways, they are fully alive with able hearts and minds. The "half person" probably will grow up to work, pay taxes, get married, worry, love a good frozen yogurt dessert, laugh, cry, and cherish with wonder the meadowlark in the backyard.

8

WOMEN AND DISABILITIES

I am not a person to take sides, particularly when it comes to my disabled brothers and sisters. However, in reviewing some statistics, the numbers concerning women with disabilities look downright discouraging. It is quite a cold shower of reality. The facts bring to fore the harsh reminders of intrinsic barriers women often face. By intrinsic barriers, I mean things like the social stigma, physical and psychological dependency, health problems, low educational achievements and the ensuing low self-esteem.

Take the social stigma. It is, in fact, responsible for so much of the pain disabled women endure. An issue that is seldom explored or even acknowledged, the social stigma is very pervasive in the lives of these women. For example, according to most data on marriage and disability, more men than women have disabilities, yet more disabled men are married, while most disabled women remain single. Numerous studies show that females who have visible physical impairments tend to remain unmarried, whereas apparent physical disabilities in men do not affect their marital status.

Too, relationships for women with disabilities are further hampered by the fact that accessibility to places, or precisely the lack thereof, tends to place the burden of getting about on the woman with a disability. The able-bodied man generally does not fare well in gracefully overcoming this obstacle with a disabled woman partner, whereas the able-bodied woman with her disabled male partner will face this task with much greater equanimity and good will.

It has also been said that the attitudes of health care providers toward the chronically ill woman may influence the quality of care she receives. For example, typical views of women may predispose physicians to attribute many of these women's symptoms to psychogenic causes. This can delay correct diagnosis and treatment of diseases that are actually of physiological origin. A classic example of this kind of misdiagnosis concerns women with AIDS. These women end up dying sooner than men who have AIDS simply because early medical intervention largely fails to take place.

And, once diagnosed with an illness, women are often subject to excessive use of unnecessary surgical techniques or mood-modifying drugs. As a result, the poor handling of women's illnesses by the medical profession may adversely affect women's abilities to adjust medically and emotionally to disabilities caused by illness.

To make matters worse, women with disabilities usually are poor. Why? One major factor is the high unemployment rate among persons with disabilities. According to a Current Population Survey (CPS), only twelve percent of women with disabilities, or one in eight, work full time. A second important factor is sex discrimination. Third, the lack of good schooling hurts — always. At best, access to higher education is difficult to obtain for almost anyone with a disability. It goes without saying, those women who have made it through obtaining higher education, disabled or not, are usually better off economically.

As far as work is concerned, the 1970s were notable for a massive movement of working-age women entering the labor force. However, most disabled women did not participate in this movement. Interestingly, according to one CPS, one working-age woman in every twelve is disabled. Yet, three out of every four disabled women of working age are out of the labor force. Sadly, despite some progress in this area, little has changed for women with disabilities. The aforementioned CPS report may be old (1981), but very little differs from year to year. To wit, the 1970 Census reported that 26 percent of working-age disabled women were in the labor force. In 1988, the figure improved slightly and stood at 27.5 percent, according to a Department of Commerce report issued in July, 1989. That is a 1.5 percent improvement over an eighteen-year span. And this 27.5 percent figure pales next to the 88.9 percent of men with no disability in the labor force.

Looking at education, we see that disabled women consistently fared worse than disabled men. For example, according to a recent CPS report, only 5.8 percent of the disabled women completed college compared to 9.1 percent of disabled men. To avoid further dismay, I dare not compare this 5.8 percent of graduating disabled women to graduating able-bodied men. Presumably, you get the picture.

Another rarely acknowledged, but equally very pervasive and weighty, problem is the violence against women with disabilities. It has been tagged as the silent epidemic. It is so silent that I had difficulty locating any statistics or organizations specifically concerning such violence. Some of the factors that contribute to the abuse of women with disabilities are similar to those affecting persons who are not disabled but are victims of abuse, such as children or elderly people. These individuals all share attributes which can include dependency, reluctance to come forward because of this very dependency, disbelief of others when told about the abuse, or inability to defend themselves because of their very situation.

Sadly, according to one researcher, Pat Murphy, a Ph.D. in the field of rehabilitation, and author of *Making the Connection: Women, Work, & Abuse* (St. Lucie Press, 1993) and *A Career & Life Planning Guide for Women Survivors: Making the Connections Workbook* (St. Lucie Press, 1996), women with disabilities, or any abused women for that matter, often share the common distress of being violated by the very persons they depend on.

The disbelief or denial of others plays an immense part in the continued silence. Today, I am both anguished and haunted by the memory of such abuse. There is an enormous price being paid. And there seems to be no end. An incalculable number of women continue to be abused as I write this. And there are untold other Bosnias, other Tibets happening right now. Meanwhile, the lack of direct networking, support groups, hot lines, and accessible shelters simply to escape the abuse, hurts. Ignorance hurts. Denial hurts. So the exploitation carries on under a wide spread shroud of continual silence. There is a saying, "God gave us shoulders so we can carry burdens." But how broad and strong do our shoulders have to be in this case?

The good news is that a majority of married women with a disability I've met have husbands who are gentle, sensitive, and very caring human beings. Almost all were in Scandinavia, where the intrinsic attitudes are less of a barrier in every respect. One picture that sticks in my mind is of Bente and Bjorn. Bente, who has quadriplegia because of a diving accident in childhood, and uses a power wheelchair, has been married to Bjorn, a chiropractor, for years. There is a photograph on their refrigerator door of the two walking the streets in Oslo. One hand of Bente's is driving her power chair; the other is holding Bjorn's hand as he walks alongside. They are both smiling.

Sponsored by the Pacific Research and Training Alliance, now called the Berkeley Planning Associates,[1] I attended the Second Annual Disabled Women's Symposium held in Oakland, California, the summer of 1995, just prior to the Society of Disability Studies (SDS)[2] convention. There were over a hundred of us from all over the country with a range of disabilities. Issues from abuse, to raising children, to developing political clout were discussed. Every culture, lifestyle, and age was represented. The theme, in fact, was "Celebrating Diversity." And diverse it was.

To get in on the ground floor of any action, you go to California, sunny beaches regardless. After years of pleading that I go to any SDS convention, on the part of the late disability activist, Kirk MacGugan, I finally went. Though Kirk's absence was acutely felt, I am glad I attended. This annual convention provides interesting and current information, fabulous networking, and a lot of plain old comfortable mingling among associates. The networking started before the convention even began. Entering an ongoing conversation midway, I heard two participants talking about a person with a disability who had successfully adopted a child. Groundbreaking news. And, because of the uniqueness of the news—which it should not be—I chimed in, "Hey, I know a person with a disability who has done that!"

The speaker asked, "Who?"

I responded by saying, "Oh, you don't know him. He lives in Stockholm, Sweden."

She turned to me and said, "Adolf Ratzka." So much for predicting a surprise.

Adolf, who has been a mentor of mine since I first knew him in 1989 (see Chapter 21), met my partner in this particular conversation, Lillian Gonzales Brown, at a workshop covering independent living issues at the World Institute on Disability (WID)[3] in 1985. The camaraderie and respect everyone shared at this workshop proved most inspiring.

And the women's symposium before the annual SDS convention was like the center of a volcano. You easily could see the swelling of its magma, molten hot and bubbling. It is close to exploding, an explosion that will be heard far and away, soon enough. To repeat, if you want to be in on the ground floor of any kind of focus and early action, you go to California. Needless to say, California is still good for something else besides its beaches.

Women with disabilities need to band together, to acknowledge our strengths, not our weaknesses, and to empower one another. We need to do this because there are a lot of obstacles before us. And the power of numbers counts here, very much. We need to make the course of our lives smoother, mostly by helping others to understand the difficulties we face. We need to do this not only for ourselves, but for our disabled daughters, and for all generations to follow. In other words, for every disabled woman, forever.

Above all, we need to recognize that disabled women of color have an added set of enormously difficult challenges. They endure a triple-disadvantaged status by the very nature of their gender, color, and being disabled. What these women endure is so unnecessary, so very wrong. Yet, the bias is perpetual against them. Just imagine having three strikes against you before you even step—or roll—outside. Just imagine.

The myth that disabled women won't—or shouldn't—have sex is a tremendous fallacy upheld by many. As a result, most women's services, such as birth control education and planning, are largely inaccessible. Start with entering a women's clinic: often times there are steps. And how often are instructions provided in alternative format for individuals who may have low vision or are blind?

Reality check? Some women may have disabilities, but regardless, all women have feelings. And most of us, disabled or not, like to love and be loved.

Reports in both Canada (via the DisAbled Women's Network, also known as DAWN)[4] and in the United States (via numerous sources) point out that when men become disabled, fifty percent of their marriages break up. For women, that figure is ninety-nine percent. What is it for women of color who are also disabled? I cannot bear the thought.

DAWN also reported at the women's conference that disabled women are twice as likely to be sexually assaulted than able-bodied women. So there is naturally a tremendous fear among disabled women to express any warmth towards others, lest it be misinterpreted. As a result, many women with disabilities are considered asexual because of their cool behavior. To make matters worse, as DAWN reported, disabled women are more likely than able-bodied women to be the victims of violence. No wonder the volcano's magma is molten hot, swelling, and about to explode.

How do we effectively channel this anger? One way is to get political. The keynote speaker was Judy Heumann, currently assistant secretary in the Office of Special Education and Rehabilitation Services of the Department of Education, appointed by President Clinton. Judy wasted no words in reminding us of the value of voter registration. These very basic words are echoes of the Dr. Martin Luther King's speeches I heard years ago. History has proven that there certainly is a resonance of truth that repeats itself.

Another basic tenet is to unite and speak up, loud and clearly. Educate others. Gently. Remember, an angry approach will tend to backfire. Also keep in mind the old adage: lack of education breeds ignorance. Sure, we are an angry and hurt people. Sure we are downtrodden and abused. Sure we are overwhelmed and tired. Sure we are often lonely and ignored. But no one lacks respect for a Trojan warrior, one who shoulders her burden with honor and pride.

9

SIGNIFICANT OTHERS
AND FRIENDS

The concern for significant others and their needs is wide-spread among persons who have disabilities. Those that share their experience may be a parent, a sibling, a husband, a wife, a lover, or a friend, to name a few. Yet, it is seldom acknowledged or addressed as a pressing issue. In ways, these significant others are a silent group. Though maybe not without sight or paralyzed from the waist down, significant others feel a lot of pain. Though not ignored, they can feel isolation. Though maybe quite mobile, they also experience barriers. Significant others also can feel a great deal of frustration, guilt, and a sense of helplessness.

One psychologist who works with couples in this situation states that a person who is the healthy, able-bodied member of the team can suffer from the disabling condition as much, if not more, than the individual with a disability. Significant others often carry these burdens silently. For example, many of us ask the healthy person, "How is _____?" instead of "How are you?" These significant others may be going through a range of feelings and may need to talk about it, not about their partner who may have a brain tumor. And such feelings are often sidestepped in discussing the latest chemotherapy treatment. The result? A harboring of unspoken feelings. In this is a silence that hurts. It can hurt the healthy significant other and it can hurt any relationship.

As an example of a better way, take Leonard and Norma. About his wife's condition, he has a marvelous attitude. He states, "Such is part of life. Norma is Norma and I still see that in her." Or take the attractive couple of Lucy and George. Their kids are college-bound. In recent years, Lucy has used a wheelchair. Does it matter to George? No. He says, "I married Lucy for love. That hasn't changed a bit."

But not everyone has been graced with such insight and understanding. It takes support. It takes space. It takes time. Significant others go through the same stages identified by Elisabeth Kübler-Ross that one experiences in the death of a loved one: denial, anger, bargaining, depression, and finally, acceptance. There is nothing wrong with these feelings, and significant others need to go through them. It is okay and important to do so. Like the old saying, "Better out in the wide world than the narrow gut."

But how many people know that? How many have been allowed the space and support to express such feelings? How many continue to field the questions about chemotherapy while not being able to talk about their own, and sometimes, very painful sorrows? "What this significant other needs is a safe environment to express their feelings, a supportive place that gives permission to do so. Others need to know it is only human to have these feelings," says the aforementioned psychologist.

I talked with many of the significant others at a retreat for couples, one partner living with a disability and the other a nondisabled individual. I asked the nondisabled member, "Where do you go," to an use an apt Stephen Levine description, "to keep your heart open in hell?" The answers ranged from church, to professional help, to the outdoors, to support groups. Several mentioned that interviews with doctors for nitty-gritty facts helped. But a couple of others described the difficulties in finding an understanding, experienced ear, especially in the medical profession.

A realization that seems to help everyone involved is that there is more to life than the world of disability. As someone once said, "Let your life be incandescent." In such trying times, it always helps to walk with a light touch and to remember that dolphins are often heard laughing.

A friend, newly disabled, was telling me how her friends were falling away. It seemed their abandonment was inexplicable, that she was doing something wrong. This brought tears to my eyes. The memory of a similar thing happening to me years ago came right back in sharp response as my friend was describing her own experience. A painful experience. Very painful. And a very lonely happening. But in ways, I am sure the situation is, was, equally painful for our friends. Watching us struggle with a new and different lifestyle, these people probably were looking at their own fear that this might happen to them, too.

Of course, it can happen. Disability is not discriminatory; people are. Those that cannot face this reality are going to have a very lonely and tough hour when their time comes. Not having fibers of strength to face differences even in others means not having much when it comes to your own personal challenge. Need I remind you of the overstated, but ever so accurate, axiom, "What goes around, comes around?"

To lose friends, as many also experience when divorcing, creates a vacuum for new friends, for a new life. For the newly disabled or divorced, this is, to look at nature, a time when the snake sheds its old skin. As with birth or death, you shed your skin alone. Becoming disabled, sadly, is a solitary experience. At such a time, of course, we need friends more than ever. It is like entering a foreign country where a new language and customs must be learned instantly. You have no choice. You cannot leave the territory. This is where you learn a lot about yourself, other people, grace, and, should I dare say, the meaning of spirituality in your life.

Written back in 1988 when first experiencing disability, my own words touch the meaning of learning something new and vastly different. I wrote,

> Life is so ironic at times, and at this juncture, I
> find myself learning to become, despite my
> increasing clumsiness, more graceful in the
> acceptance of such twists and changes.

Many, many people speak, and have spoken so for centuries, about the importance and value of learning to accept what any experience may have to teach you, disabled or not. Jack Kornfield, in his book, *Seeking the Heart of Wisdom,* says,

> The quality of acceptance is the ground out of
> which true insight and understanding develop.
> If we don't accept some aspect of ourselves — a
> feeling, a physical or mental sense of ourselves —
> then we cannot learn about it. We cannot
> discover its nature and become free in relation-
> ship to it. We become afraid, we resist, we judge,
> and we try to push away. We cannot look deeply
> and push away at the same time. When mind-
> fulness is well developed and the ground of
> acceptance is laid, then the body and mind are
> filled with a sense of comfort.

Dr. Carol Gill, a psychologist specializing in disability issues, addresses the very apprehension of those turning away by saying,

> Severely [or not so severely] disabled people are
> an affront to those who cannot handle any
> bumps in the human landscape. Many people
> fear our needs and worry that they may someday
> share our fate. They associate disability with
> inescapable suffering and helplessness — loss of
> control over life. They lack the imagination to
> see that a person could be paralyzed or use a
> respirator and still have an immensely valuable
> life that he or she manages, with or without
> assistance, in creative ways.

Interestingly, for me, and probably for many other people now living with a disability, this so-called "tragedy" has been the best thing that has ever happened. I, like many others, would not change a thing. With the shedding of the old skin, I like what I now see and feel. But that took a while. No doubt about it. So what helped me during the tough times? Zane Grey's words:

> To bear up under loss, to fight the bitterness of defeat and the weakness of grief, to be victor over anger, to smile when tears are close, to resist evil men and base instincts, to hate hate and to love love, to go on when it would seem good to die, to seek ever after the glory and the dream, to look up with unquenchable faith in something evermore about to be, that is what any man can do, and so be great.

10

EDUCATION

A friend once said, "Education costs less than ignorance." How very true — in more ways than one. Education is a ticket to freedom. Educated people not only have a higher income, but enjoy a fuller, and more independent, life. Unfortunately, the opposite is also true.

Lack of education keeps many submerged in the quagmire of ignorance, of dependency, of an endless round of misery. Too, lack of education hurts. According to a 1989 Current Population Studies (CPS) report by the Department of Commerce, persons who have completed less than eight years of school have a disability rate that is more than three times as high as the rate for high school graduates and eight times the rate for college graduates. Years later, there is no reason to believe this painfully apparent statistic has changed. That it most likely remains the same, or worse, merely underscores the truth.

But ignorance does not just affect those who drop out of school. Ignorance falls on *all* of our shoulders. For example, lack of education means increased tax dollars to support those who need aid in supporting themselves. So it helps to realize how education saves us money in the long run. There are many ways in which this occurs. For example, take the AIDS epidemic. The consensus is that education can be one of its greatest deterrents.

For persons with disabilities, education can mean an increased chance of employment. To wit, the 1989 CPS report further states that there is a major correlation between years of school completed and employment: they both increase proportionally. It goes without saying, of course, that increased employment means increased income. For those with disabilities, added income can mean the ability to hire extra help. Hiring extra help where we live can mean staying out of an expensive nursing home. Too, when individuals lack the resources, nursing homes are often paid by Medicare or Medicaid. These bills are handled by our state and federal taxes. And who pays for that?

Fortunately, a refreshing change is finally happening in our schools. Young people with special needs are becoming more and more integrated into the standard classroom. This is partly due to good, insightful, innovative people working in the field. Also, it is due to parents of young children with disabilities who do not want their children in special, but separate, classrooms and have been — or are becoming — more vocal about the matter. It is partly due to very specific amendments to the law commonly known as the Individuals with Disabilities Education Act (IDEAS). And, of course, the ADA has played its part.

The practice of separating students with different needs into "special" classrooms and programs has really been damaging in the long run. This is because many teachers in the field of special education, excellent and committed though they may be, tend to have low expectations of their students. These expectations have contributed to students' lower self-esteem, have increased their drop-out rate, and have seldom encouraged them to reach their true potential, including attending college. Numerous studies and case histories have shown that the participating students' skills would actually improve when they were included in a standard classroom.

Because of the higher expectations in standard classes, these students work on rising to the level of their nondisabled peers. And, not surprisingly, many succeed.

As a point we can learn from our Canadian neighbors, Judith Snow said at a conference on school inclusion held years ago,

> Those who are members of society and those who are marginalized from society have a great need for each other's gifts . . . if they [persons with disabilities] are brought back into the arms of society, they become the architects of the new community; a community that has a new capacity to support everyone's needs and inter-actions.

Take Mark Medoff, author, playwright, and teacher known nationally for writing the play, *Children of a Lesser God.* He has found working with kids who have disabilities, from very diverse backgrounds, a most gratifying experience. He has been involved in developing a new play called *Another Planet.* Working with mid-level students, their parents, teachers, and other community members, Mark talks about watching the participants evolve and bond. He says, "In three short weeks, I began to see a change. Kids from very different abilities and backgrounds began to see what similarities they did have. They have developed friendships and have continued to grow, evolve, and share."

But the movement toward inclusion certainly does not mean we are all the same. Nor does it mean there is a consensus, that we all agree. Rather, moving toward inclusion means moving toward acceptance of our differences with respect. It means supporting each other, regardless. It is also an antidote to racism and sexism because it welcomes all differences and celebrates them as capacities rather then deficiencies. Starting early in school, children's perception of what is normal or ordinary becomes altered in a good way. Children learn, at a very young age, about diversity and difference. They learn that there is no such thing as "normal."

I attended a conference involving Jack Pearpoint, Marsha
Forest of the Centre for Integrated Education and Community[1] in Toronto, Canada, and Dr. Mary Falvey, a professor at
California State University/Los Angeles, School of Education.[2] The conference primarily dealt with the nitty-gritty of
integrating students with disabilities into the regular classroom. On a subject known more as "inclusion" within educational circles, this conference was predominately attended by
school administrators, teachers, concerned parents, and physical or occupational therapists, all strong believers and propo-
nents of inclusion in our schools and communities. We
attendees were anxious to learn the details of how to make
equal learning work in our schools.

Just what does inclusion mean? According to Pearpoint
and Forest, a good definition of inclusion is *with*, students
going to classes with students, disabled or not. None of this
special and separate stuff for "students with special needs."
Separate is simply considered unequal. Jack and Marsha point
out inclusion means "in" as the term "inclusion," or "to include," implies. Genuine learning occurs among students side
by side, disabled or not. In fact, true learning happens with
any of us, anywhere, anytime, in school or in a neighborhood
meeting together, en masse, side-by-side. In the inclusive
classroom, there grows a sense of fellowship among all. The
students practice " . . . cooperation, not competition; participation, not coercion; relationships, not isolation; interdepen-
dence, not independence; friendships, not isolation," according
to Marsha and Jack.

I spoke with Leau Phillips, co-executive director with Cindy
White of Inclusion New Mexico! Leau says, "Inclusion means
more than just tolerating. It means celebrating one another
and our differences while remembering we are more alike than
different."

Patricia Mullen, a conference participant and long-time
inclusion advocate, recounts the story Pearpoint and Forest
told when she first met them back in 1987. Pearpoint and
Forest were describing one of the negative effects of not practicing inclusion, of keeping kids in separate classrooms. They

used the analogy of a child and its companion, a pet dog. The dog gets hit by a car and dies. And what does the child learn in school the next few days? Nothing. Being so isolated by grief, the child hurts, badly. Likewise, being so isolated in a separate classroom, the child with "special needs" hurts, badly.

Put a child with cerebral palsy (CP) into a regular classroom with fellow classmates and everyone learns. As with all the students, the same high standards of performance are expected of the child with CP. Because of such expectations, this student naturally does better. Meanwhile, the other students learn about compassion, care, and the genuineness of equal existence. You know, the side-by-side stuff.

Think about it. Don't we adults do better when our bosses expect more of us? And don't we all express tenderness when helping out an infant? Who benefits? Everyone. Absolutely everyone. It is that natural, that symbiotic. Like the saying, "Practice faith and there is more around," so goes inclusion. Exercise inclusion and there is more inclusion that will take place, naturally. More than anything, it is a way of thinking. They say, "Attitude is the true disability." How true. Watching videos and hearing stories at the conference really brought this home, again and again. But inclusion is more than just an academic thought. Include young folks with any kind of disability in our lives, and they learn about relationships, socialization, and responsibility as well.

Such skills are vital to any young person who is to make the transition from the classroom to the "real" world out there. In the evening hours, there was a great deal of discussion about this pressing issue among the conference participants. At best, any transition is problematic. For the child to learn the tools of daily survival is a critical concern of any parent, particularly if the child is grappling with a disability in addition to the everyday stuff.

Take this a step further. Learning about friendship? Sexuality? Parenting? It's not easy. I spoke about this very dilemma with Pruda Trujillo, a conference participant, a special education teacher, and mother of a son who is developmentally delayed. How is she to discuss all this with him? Who makes the decisions? There are no easy answers. Meanwhile, our children are growing up. And there is no time.

Even over forty years ago, Earl Warren, then chief justice of the U.S. Supreme Court, stipulated in a May 17, 1954, case:

> Separate educational facilities are inherently
> unequal. This inherent inequality stems from
> the stigma created by purposeful segregation
> which generates a feeling of inferiority that may
> affect their hearts and minds in a way unlikely
> ever to be undone.

Forty years ago. And have we really seen any progress? For anyone? Any situation? Any place? I ask myself again. And ask others.

Deb Wilson, who has a job working for the Albuquerque Public School system and is currently in the University of New Mexico's Communicative Disorder department, says, "Given the proper support, inclusion works. And it has tremendous potential." Deb should know. Previously, she worked for an organization whose primary focus was to see that children with disabilities were experiencing inclusion at the community level. Logic says, if we can do it at the community level, why not in the schools? And is not education an integral, vital spoke in the wheel of life, of basic community involvement, of societal responsibility?

Meanwhile, Dr. Mary Falvey, a widely published author, activist, and designer of programs for teachers, researchers, and leaders facilitating inclusion, offers nuts and bolts solutions for making sure inclusion works. Mary provides an overview of assessment, curriculum, and instruction for inclusive classes. Her day-to-day practicum relates to Earl Warren's words of forty years ago. She offers the following suggestions for creating inclusion among all students in all classrooms, and for structuring the classroom environment. She says:

- Establish a "classroom community" or a "caring community."

- Provide a place to help facilitate a sense of community among the students to improve self-esteem and a sense of belonging.

- Create an atmosphere of trust.

- Let it be a place where clear expectations, goals, and learning outcomes are shared.

- Emphasize cooperation rather than competition.

- Provide an atmosphere where the teacher's authenticity, nonjudgmental attitude, fairness, and congruent communication to students can flourish.

Dr. Falvey suggests that a democratic classroom can be created by providing a place where:

- Choices are clear.

- Discipline is logical.

- Self-discipline is encouraged.

- The most positive components of a democratic society are mirrored.

She encourages schools to follow four plans of action in creating a democratic classroom.

- Establish a climate of mutuality and respect.

- Encourage students.

- Offer students roles in decision making.

- Develop students' self-discipline through consistent, logical, fully understood guidelines for their behavior.

Dr. Falvey is a beacon of light for youngsters with disabilities. She makes inclusion happen in our schools. We need a Dr. Mary Falvey. Everywhere. At all times. Period.

Obviously, a teacher cannot do all the above alone. Simply, that is asking too much. We must provide the teacher with support to see that inclusion can be accomplished, much as worker bees do for their queen bee to ensure the production of honey. After all, inclusion is a very sweet affair.

Along with hiring aides, we can offer extra credit for a student to be a "classroom companion" to one in need of extra help. Ask parents or college-level or graduate students or volunteers to stop in one to three times a week to monitor and help foster further cooperation among all.

In other words, there are ways to draw the community in to create the "classroom community." Meet together one or two times a month. Be an active community in the classroom. Obviously, it's a win-win deal: better classrooms, better students, a better community, a better world. Then ask, is progress being made?

I think about all the young folks who are severely injured in car accidents and end up becoming wheelchair users, and then some, as a result. Sad as this may be, it is no surprise. According to the National Spinal Cord Injury Association (SCI), a nonprofit organization for individuals living with spinal cord injury (phone: 1-800-962-9629), their families, friends, and related professionals, the most frequent age at injury is nineteen.

It is also stated in one of their 1996 fact sheets that motor vehicle accidents are the leading cause of SCI (forty-four percent), followed by acts of violence (twenty-four percent), falls (twenty-two percent), sports (eight percent), and then, other things (two percent). It is interesting to also note that ninety-two percent of all sports injuries result in quadriplegia. Again, no surprise—just think of Christopher Reeve. His situation upholds both of the oft-said axioms, "Disability is a club anyone can join," and "People with paraplegia are born, while people with quadriplegia are made."

I was talking to a woman I know in the publishing field, Emily, and asked about her husband's student, Adriana, who now uses a wheelchair as a result of a car accident at the end of her sophomore year in high school. Emily and I got to talking about Adriana's future, whether or not she goes on to college. But, the "to-be-or-not-to-be" question is a waste of time. That should not even be a question. Whether you walk or roll, see or don't see, hear or do not hear, should absolutely have no bearing on any possible future plans. Granted, going to school may take longer for Adriana, but education is a right, everyone's right, according to the law.

High school is a crummy time to be injured. It's just when we are getting to know ourselves better, testing trust, placing stock into our personalities and others, figuring out about life, sex, dating, college, and much more. To be considered different in any way is, but should not be, the way peers in high school judge one another. Harsh. Cruel. And then some. There are so many unknowns being faced then. It not only takes an act of courage in dealing with added difficulties, it takes courage on anyone's part to merely face reality, period. This reminds me of a poignant song, "Courage," written by Bob Blue, an elementary school teacher and composer living in Massachusetts.

> A small thing once happened at school
> That brought up a question for me,
> And somehow, it forced me to see
> The price that I pay to be cool.
> Diane is a girl that I know.
> She's strange, like she doesn't belong.
> I don't mean to say that that's wrong,
> We don't like to be with her, though.
> And so when we all made a plan
> To have this big party at Sue's,
> Most kids in school got the news,
> But no one invited Diane.
> The thing about Taft Junior High,
> Is secrets don't last very long.
> I acted like nothing was wrong
> When I saw Diane start to cry.
> I know you may think that I'm cruel.
> It doesn't make me very proud.
> I just went along with the crowd.

It's sad, but you have to at school.
You fit in as well as you can.
I couldn't be friends with Diane,
Cause then they would treat me like her.
In one class at Taft Junior High,
We study what people have done
With gas chamber, bomber and gun
In Auschwitz, Japan, and My Lai.
I don't understand all I learn.
Sometimes I just sit there and cry.
The whole world stood idly by
To watch as the innocent burned.
Like robots obeying some rule.
Atrocities done by the mob.
All innocents, doing their job.
And what was it for? Was it cool?
The world was aware of this hell,
But how many cried out in shame?
No heroes, nobody to blame.
A story that no one dared to tell.
I promise to do what I can
To not let it happen again.
To care for all women and men.
I'll start by inviting Diane.

College? Go, Adriana, go.

11

ACCESSIBLE HOUSING

In Scandinavian countries and Canada, it is already well-established that every member of their communities will have difficulty encountering the built environment sometime during their lifetime. Their attitude is that the needs of those who face various kinds of functional challenges are to be accepted as part of the norm. This includes a far larger sector than just those with disabilities. Consider elderly people, pregnant women, individuals who are temporarily infirm, those who are injured, and infants, to name a few. Accessible, safe, and adaptable homes are designed for up to fifty-five percent of the population at one time if you include all the aforementioned. This is a scope far larger than the estimated, and growing, twenty percent of America's population with disabilities.

In the past, traditional thinking has resulted in the design and construction of dwellings with emphasis on "the structure"—its appearance, construction methods, and materials and emphasis on "the normal man"—which is realistically a very small percentage of the population at any given time. But genuine consideration for safety, ease of use, adaptability, and costs for the whole spectrum of social application is, fortunately, gaining priority on the planner's and designer's checklist.

If we are to take seriously the goal that all dwellings should be for all people at all times, then all buildings must be designed precisely with that in mind, beginning with the architect's initial conceptual drawings. As repeatedly stated by related professionals, the cost of doing so runs only one to two percent more if done at the drawing board stage. In other words, it is to be treated as foresight, not hindsight.

There are some decisive qualities which, without pushing costs beyond the normal level, easily could be incorporated into present-day construction. It is a matter of built-in practicality, of thoughtful spatial standards, of lifestyle awareness, and of communication among designers, architects, builders, developers, therapists, politicians, and, of course, users/occupants.

Accessibility is now so ingrained into the social structure and lifestyles, mores, laws, and financial situation of the aforementioned countries that their design solutions to dwellings are for the present *as well as* for the future. In other words, these countries now design dwellings for all people at all times. This is demonstrably good sense. As a result, most recently built dwellings there are functional, flexible, and cherished homes where everyone can continue to live their lives through many years. The designs allow for any change of, or among, user/occupant without creating exorbitant remodeling costs. Also, by such designs, unnecessary lengthy hospital stays due to accidents are equally alleviated.

I came to discover that barrier-free design does not mean institutional-appearing, and produces easy and pleasant environments. It was wonderful to witness the simplicity and unobtrusiveness of such design solutions. Most sites I visited offered the ambiance of lightness and spaciousness with white walls, light oak floors, wide doors and hallways, and a minimum amount of clutter. The touches of warmth necessary because of dark winter days in these northerly latitudes were added with good use of plants, light furniture colors, and excellent indoor lighting, both artificial and natural.

In recent years, efforts have increased to make public buildings and transportation accessible to people with disabilities in the United States. Fortunately this is changing, albeit slowly, due to the efforts of the federal government. It only makes sense, then, that accessible housing will follow suit. Sadly, accessible housing issues are slow to be recognized here in the United States, largely because building codes and laws affecting dwellings do not make accessibility a requirement.

Not only do individuals with disabilities need to know about these design alternatives, but architects, builders, developers, and other users can benefit from such knowledge. Instead of designing a "special" place accommodating "special" individuals, aesthetic incorporation of such accommodations means absorption into mainstream design, creating homes for all people, in all ways, at all times. It means concurrent use by a mixed population with varying needs and a normalizing of social activities, something we all cherish. And when accomplished at the drawing board stage, well before any need of a jackhammer to rectify, it means minimal additional costs.

For architects, builders, and developers, awareness means lower costs at time of construction. Consider the following "what-if" scenario presented by architect Ellen Harland eight years ago. The cost to install a two-foot, eight-inch door during the normal course of new construction would be approximately $610. If it became apparent at the design stage that the code required a three-foot-wide door and a different type of hardware, the increase in cost would be a mere $10 or $15 — the cost of a wider door. Had the door already been installed and work essentially complete, the jackhammer correction would cost an additional $772. And these costs were computed in 1988. Such foresight is worth even more today.

Currently, there are 50 million Americans with disabilities, a little more than twenty percent of the population, many of whom are looking for work and places to live independently. With increased rehabilitation, retraining, and laws that require both the education and employment of persons with disabilities, an increasing number of individuals with disabilities will be entering the work force. And, of course, they'll need places to live. Too, our population is aging, and better house design can alleviate the need to reside in nursing homes during our later years.

Upon research years ago, well before the signing of the Americans with Disabilities Act, I found that in countries with some form of socialized programs, such as in Canada, Sweden, Denmark, and Norway, the policies of housing persons with disabilities and the elderly in their own homes had proven to be less costly (by one-half) than housing—or as the saying goes here, "warehousing"—anyone in an institution. These countries struggle with their burgeoning social responsibilities as their population, like that of America, ages. Consequently, they are very proactive in attempts to find both tangible and intangible solutions.

In Sweden alone, between a quarter and a third of the adult population is either disabled or over the age of sixty-five. As a result, since 1977, Swedish building laws have required that not only public premises, but also all new and renovated homes must be accessible to persons in wheelchairs or with any other disability. This is one attempt at a clearly stated goal: to save taxes. Scandinavian people reason that senior citizens and persons with disabilities should be able to stay in their homes and receive help and care in their familiar environment instead of residing in any costly and strange institution.

For cost reasons alone, Denmark decided to phase out almost all of its nursing homes. So where does everyone go now? Current master planning of new quarters includes mixed living complexes ranging from single-person apartments to family or group homes. These government-subsidized projects primarily house, among the general population, children, families, attendants, elderly folks, and individuals with disabilities. As far back as 1988, social housing in Denmark comprised eighteen percent of all housing and forty-five percent of all rental units. Undoubtedly, these figures have increased today with a flourishing graying population.

It has also been the basic policy of the Scandinavian countries to recognize persons with disabilities as a social minority entitled to equal housing opportunity and daily living assistance. As quoted from the Swedish Institute's 1989 fact sheet on "Support for the Handicapped in Sweden,"

> Construction of new buildings or extensive renovations are required to take the needs of mobility and orientationally impaired individuals in mind. With these efforts in accessible design, most handicapped [sic] individuals are able to live in normal modern buildings.

Continuing to quote from this fact sheet, the Swedish philosophy suggests a proactive approach:

> The objective of Swedish housing policy is to provide the whole population with sound, well-planned and practical dwellings of a high standard and at a reasonable cost. In planning housing, special regard should be paid to the needs of the elderly and the handicapped [sic]. Experience shows that, with good basic planning according to the guidelines stated in the building by-laws, it is possible to achieve such a high degree of accessibility that the majority of handicapped persons [sic] can manage in a normal modern dwelling.

Norway, Denmark, and Canada are following Swedish policies, Sweden being a country whose social welfare and medical care programs go back as far as the sixteenth century. These other countries are aware of the economic, social, and political implications of mainstreaming home design for individuals with disabilities as well as any elderly person.

The Swedish housing journalist, Ollie Bengtzon, takes the concept a step further by stating:

> Conscious home-consumers are demanding aesthetic qualities to an ever increasing extent... and both housing owners and contractors are becoming aware that beauty can also be an important function.

Kerstin Wickman, then editor-in-chief of Sweden's leading design magazine, *Form,* and lecturer at the National College of Art and Design, says that recent Swedish design trends include "honesty, sensuousness, insight, and genuineness . . ." Lennart Lindkvist, director of the Swedish Society of Crafts and Design, continues the thought by saying, "It is said that a nation's design is a reflection of its society; there is no doubt that the design of everyday objects presents a picture of our ordinary culture and lifestyles." The Japanese also reflect this in their standards for quality: a commitment to tiny improvements in a thousand places.

The Scandinavian treatment of accessibility reflects their social philosophy in their newer buildings by de-institutionalizing the accommodation of special needs. This is particularly noted in kitchen design and technology, an area of necessary function and social activity among all.

Too, current Norwegian thought treats disability as a normal phenomenon. As a result, developing ordinary housing layout standards to include "Life Span Dwellings" is a recommended solution. A Life Span Dwelling, according to architect Tore Lange, is a structure where all activities can occur on one floor without necessitating the use of stairs.

Scandinavian design traditions reveal principles dictating both aesthetics and function. Because of laws addressing increasing social needs, these concerns spill over into the treatment of independence and lifestyle leading to increased grace and normalization of "the differently-abled population" into their mainstream.

Some Practical Reasoning

A Homelink coordinator for the London, Ontario March of Dimes chapter reinforced the idea that an accessible home will be a salable home, especially in large, crowded metropolitan areas such as Toronto. He stated, "We've been doing an analysis of housing, and [have found] a lot of housing is in apartments, so it doesn't leave a lot of options. Townhouses are also a problem because there are upstairs bedrooms. So we're trying to convince developers to build more accessible housing."[1]

That is *integrated* accessible housing. Integration is so necessary to avoid the "special" clustering of such homes or apartments that may carry with it the stigma of a "special" population. As a result of this thinking, the Swedish Folkus Flats, a series of special, accessible apartments built in the seventies, are now found to be segregating in their appearance, and are no longer appreciated. Unfortunately, other communities in Europe followed suit to the Folkus Flats. These places are now referred to as "golden ghettoes" because of their segregating nature.

Many of us unexpectedly become disabled or have an aging parent who needs to stay with us to recover from a broken hip or stroke. The old rhetoric, disability is a club *anyone* can join at *any time* is, unfortunately, still ever so true. Under such circumstances, to continue living where we have been living becomes of added importance for psychological and financial reasons. And the concept of integrating accessible homes in the community allows for the increased acceptance of persons with disabilities and elderly individuals.

Costs

Repeatedly, I met architect after architect overseas, who stated that building a barrier-free home from scratch added, perhaps, one percent of the total cost, and at the most, two percent. One percent is incurred by the need of larger spaces, such as four-foot-wide hallways and wider doors. Two percent is for added special equipment, such as the pneumatic kitchen counters or built-in ceiling lifts.

In considering these modest increases, Dr. Adolf Ratzka, once a research economist at Stockholm's School of Architecture, Institute of Technology, feels that once a structure is accessible, it will remain so and yield both tangible and intangible cost benefits throughout its existence. For example, he states that one tangible benefit will include savings to the individual and the public in form of fewer accidents because of the enhanced safety that comes with accessible design. The result is less need for subsequent long-term hospitalization.

In the same study, however (*The Costs of Disabling Environments*),[2] Dr. Ratzka found that if all costs and benefits are considered, it is even economical to retrofit old structures with elevators even when these buildings have as few as three floors and only nine apartments per elevator.

Meanwhile, the Norwegians are trying officially to develop the Life Span Dwelling concept, where a living room, a kitchen, a shower and toilet, and at least one bedroom are on the main floor, fully and easily accessible. Because it is assumed that the incorporation of this concept to the normal standard of housing would pay in the long run, the Norwegian State Housing Bank has offered reduced loans for those who follow the prescriptions of Life Span Dwellings.

With newer technology entering the private accessible home market, such as pneumatic kitchen counters, communication systems, and ergonomic hand tools for daily living, costs drop for personal care and attendant care. As far back as ten years ago, Gini Laurie reported in her monograph, *European Concepts of Independent Living:*[3]

> The Davises kept track of how much help they needed per week for the two of them. When they were in an institution, they needed $33\frac{1}{2}$ hours per week. In the first week in their new flat, they needed 8 hours. By the third month, it was 4 hours, and now, it is $1\frac{1}{2}$ hours.

In this same monograph, Ms. Laurie continued:

> The United Kingdom studies estimate that only two percent of the disabled might need special housing and that ninety-eight percent of the disabled could use "mobility housing"—that is, housing with accessible entrances and essential movement throughout.

Taking the above rationale into consideration, plus an aging population, plus increasing social burdens, the argument of high building costs for any special-needs population is no longer valid.

Hanne Weiss-Lindencrona, once involved in Sweden's Ministry of Housing and Physical Planning, says,

> Often, it is what people *imagine* [author's emphasis] the costs to be that is the biggest obstacle. We must put an end to the myth that accessibility results in high building costs.

She reiterates the intangible, and hard-to-measure, values:

> . . . how to evaluate the gains of the individual in terms of personal integrity, self-respect, feeling of security or maintained social networks? These benefits are some of the reasons behind the desire for a home of one's own and to keep it as long as one wishes."[4]

To sum up, what you generally witness in these countries is the success of their governmental approaches and practical solutions to the aforementioned challenge. In other words, you are looking at, not necessarily "where the grass is greener," but where a form of socialized government works.

Safety

Looking at safety in any kind of dwelling, statistics disclose that tripping and falling cause far more deaths than such emergencies as fires and earthquakes. "To be exact, they cause six times more deaths," according to Clara Yoshida in her report, *Three Stage Housing for Old People.*[5] Another survey on the occurrence of these accidents points out that they mainly happen at entrances, on the floor, and on staircases. The largest cause of tripping and/or falling is encounters with floor sills, floor level changes, steps, and loose rugs.

Dr. Adolf Ratzka, in his report mentioned above, *The Costs of Disabling Environments,* stipulates that in Sweden, accidents involving a fall account for twice as many disabilities as those incurred in traffic circumstances. He also points out that a disproportionate number of elderly people are exposed to this kind of accident and up to ten percent of all these accidents involve falls on staircases.

As the Norwegian architect Tore Lange stresses, the safety advantages of living in Life Span Dwellings are largely that there are no staircases in such design. Other design features that address safety issues, and yet continue to maintain a mainstream appearance with no or little additional cost, include elimination of floor level changes and door sills. Bare, light-colored hardwood floors are very popular because of their appearance, smoothness, resilience (as compared to tile and/or brick), and ease in cleaning. Good lighting, both natural and artificial, contributes to enhanced safety. This lighting is built in, either via skylights, well-placed windows, or lights on the walls and/or on the ceilings, thereby eliminating dangerous cords and any clutter.

Psychological Values

The late disability-rights advocate, Dr. Kirk MacGugan of New Mexico, said,

> Many of us are categorized as needing sterile
> and hospital-like accessibility, when what we
> really desire is architectural design to catch up
> with the independent living movement. We
> want the spaces we live in to be comfortable,
> beautiful, and relaxing.

Too, it is a well-known axiom that people do better if they continue to be physically and intellectually active on all levels. This contributes to our wholeness, both individually and within our society. Everyone—the able-bodied and individuals with disabilities—benefits by such integrity. Since our work and living spaces can be manipulated to remain most viable with respect to our needs, the retrofitting of dwellings can serve to eliminate relocation to a strange and, most likely, debilitating environment. Sadly, persons with disabilities and the elderly will tolerate a great deal to remain in familiar home environments and neighborhoods. To force them into this kind of tolerance is an unnecessary act on our part.

Needless to say, there is a great psychological benefit when the environment has been designed with a holistic approach providing the necessary freedom of movement and allowing for all activities, adding to the user's self-determination, independence, and contribution to society. Too, an individual's psychological well-being is an immeasurable, integrated thread in the web of society's well-being.

Though intangible in terms of economic benefits, there are other costs to be paid if the psychological benefits are ignored. To quote Dr. Ratzka's report, *The Costs of Disabling Environments:*

> The prospect of life in segregated facilities is a powerful incentive for many disabled persons to hold out in inaccessible environments at the price of physical overexertion, risk of accidents, and premature loss of functional abilities. The impact of inaccessible environments on the personality development of children and adults, their self-image as environmentally incompetent persons and on the attitudes of the general population towards such "helpless" people have been studied very little. The physical and mental energy spent on coping with our inaccessible cities, the imposed restrictions in lifestyle, occupational and social opportunities, are again costs born not only by disabled people, their families and friends, but by us all.

Another solution in creating accessible, integrated communities involves cohousing.[6] A concept born in Denmark, it is now realizing growth here in North America including Canada.

Cohousing. What is it? Briefly, a group of people, all ages, all kinds, collectively organize, plan, buy acreage, and build a cluster of homes in which to live together. Throw in a few wonderful amenities such as a plaza, a common community center, and surrounding individuals that care about you.

Cohousing. It's one alternative answer by today's baby boom generation to our "last stop," among other social ills. Cohousing is a way back to our communities. Says WindSong Cohousing member, Laurie Usher, "I am interested in cohousing for a sense of closeness and the process of consciously choosing how I want to live."

A cohousing group, usually organized a minimum of five years before actually moving into their newly-built residences, plans everything. They even choose their architect and have a very active say in the design of the buildings. This group also determines things such as the philosophy of their ideals and choosing how they will operate living together as a loosely-knit extended family. And they can determine just how accessible their place will be. Thus, a five-year gestation period occurs before they even realize the birth of their efforts. As with anything good, it takes a lot of hard work and tremendous commitment to make this happen.

Each cohousing unit is different. What cohousing groups usually share in common is a vehicle-free courtyard, akin to the plazas so prevalent in states like New Mexico and in countries like Italy. Plazas are a conducive space where anyone can visit, play, garden or simply be. Vehicle-free plazas are considered safe environments. All parking and other vehicular traffic takes place on the periphery of the housing cluster. In other words, the back door and garage face the outer circle of the homes. Again, in the center of the circle is the protected, traffic-free plaza, easily observed from most of the individual homes nearby. The other shared thing cohousing arrangements usually provide is a common dining/meeting hall where one can join in a community meal. Or instead, members can choose to cook and eat in the quiet of their own home. Miriam Evers of WindSong comments on the value of the community eating hall by saying, ". . . and the thought of not having to cook every night . . ." Within this community hall are usually a children's playroom and laundry room as well. Whether they use the facilities or not, every member of the cohousing group contributes financially to the building costs of this common hall.

Cohousing. It is a way of caring for each other. Say other WindSong members about why they have chosen to live in a cohousing arrangement, ". . . a desire to create an extended family . . . where people know and help each other . . . to grow old with [these] people around . . ."

Again, this marvelous way of living originates from Denmark. And people with disabilities benefit largely from this thoughtful arrangement. How? The obvious factor is the elimination of isolation. There is no cumbersome transportation hassle about visiting your community of importance. You simply go to the nearby inner courtyard or the common dining hall—rain, snow, or whatever. Also, you can hire one or more individuals from this community to be your attendant(s) for daily activity and/or long-term caretakers. That is a win-win situation for everyone involved. How? Parents can work within walking distance of their own home, sharing flex-time with the other hired attendants within the community. Job sharing. A dream of many. And to work within a home environment—a dream of equally many. That there is less job commuting means less air pollution and less ozone depletion in addition. This is another win-win situation. For whom? For you and me, disabled or not, and the world.

There also is the intrinsic value of children being around a person with a disability. These children grow up with the realization that we are all naturally different. And, chances are, these children will be their natural selves among all of us different folks. Who wins? Society.

CHAPTER

12

TRANSPORTATION

A basic need in this mobile, sprawling city where I live is a way to get around. In other words, some wheels are necessary. Some of us drive, some take the bus, some ride a bike, and a few even walk. But persons with disabilities seldom have such choices. Yes, there is a special bus system for persons with disabilities; but no, you can't go out for a spontaneous cup of coffee with friends at the Double Rainbow, a great coffee joint and bakery. Why? You need to call at least twenty-four hours ahead of time to schedule your ride on the special transit system. With such planning and programming required beforehand, all spontaneity is lost.

As our city grows, naturally there will be more Double Rainbows. And naturally, there will be more persons with disabilities. Equally, we all desire to be involved in our city's life one way or another, disabled or not. Yet, we do not necessarily like to book transportation twenty-four hours prior any more than we like to experience air pollution. But that seems to be the city's plan for the future by maintaining this special, and separate, transportation system for those in need. Of course, there is increased pollution because of these additional vehicles running around. And of course, there is an increased tax burden for everyone in order to maintain this special but separate transportation system.

Transportation is a vital link that brings people together for work, recreation, daily activities, and more. Accessible transportation opens the door to independence for both persons with disabilities and seniors, the two sectors of our population that tend to be greatly isolated by the lack of such amenity. Creating a unified, accessible public transportation system is a win-win situation all around. In utilizing such a system, persons with disabilities become integrated, functional members of society. They can be tax payers instead of tax recipients for the simple reason that they can get to work in a timely and cost-effective manner. Equally, society in general can interact more casually with persons who have disabilities. In doing so, we not only become more familiar with various disabilities, but can also find mingling on the job, in the library, or in the store that much easier. Such added familiarization increases anyone's comfort level. Comfort is one of the biggest eliminators of the misunderstandings, attitudinal bias, and patronizing behavior that so commonly occur in unfamiliar situations. And for all, by using public transit, we will see less automobile pollution, fewer traffic gridlocks, and fewer barrels earmarking the ubiquitous repair jobs and endless road construction.

And as our population grows older, more and more aging, but basically able-bodied, people are going to use these wonderful three-wheel scooters (what I call my "motorized rickshaw") to get around the mall with their hip crumbling, knee out of commission, or with added difficulty in breathing. Too, rickshaws are certainly one way of keeping up with speedy grandkids.

Accessible public transportation can be an excellent solution to our mobility needs. But, as most of us realize, public transit systems are painfully slow in accommodating us despite ADA (Americans with Disabilities Act) mandates here. Privately-owned paratransit systems are no better as a solution.

So there is much we can learn much about accessible transportation systems from our Canadian neighbors and Swedish counterparts. Because Canada's population is aging like ours, fewer and fewer people will be driving there in the future, due to increasing disabilities that come naturally with age, the desire not to drive anymore, finances, or simply the wish to live a simpler lifestyle. Yet, Canada doesn't have a government mandate requiring accessible public transportation. Simply, the people there have found it more cost-effective, less polluting, and more enjoyable to make public transportation readily accessible. A grandmother, disabled or not, can take her grandchild to the zoo with minimal effort. A person with a disability can ride along with a friend carrying on their sociable—and in many cases, endless — dialogue en route.

Because Canada understands the use of and importance of public transportation for all, its national strategy underlines the principle that persons with disabilities should be able to travel with the same ease and dignity as others. For example, take the city of Vancouver. Getting around Greater Vancouver on public transit has never been easier for persons with disabilities. You have a wide variety of options, regardless of whether you use a wheelchair or a three-wheel scooter, or have a disability that makes climbing stairs difficult. For most riders, reduced fares are available on all modes of travel, whether it is a bus, a taxi, the light rail system, or the ferry, encouraging greater use by the citizens. Too, every transit operator is well trained in offering services to individuals with any kind of special need. Equally, most of the Vancouver buses and taxis have lifts big enough to accommodate individuals who use three-wheel scooters, not a common design practice here in America.

Because Vancouver's transit system organization has worked closely with advocacy groups that promote accessible, public transportation for persons with disabilities, their system is considered one of the most progressive in all of North America. It is a cost-effective alternative to the special, and separate, transit systems found so commonly in the United

States. A well-mixed, well-utilized public transportation system pollutes less, costs less, and certainly promotes greater integration of persons with disabilities into mainstream society as well.

13

RECREATION
AND LEISURE

Summertime. Gardens emerge, trees produce. The ballads of the cicadas surge and fade. Convertibles become topless. Children splash away hot afternoons. We walk or roll more slowly. And it's not too hard to emulate a dog's pattern of an afternoon siesta. It is all cotton dress and shorts. Even if you work full-time, have ten kids, and fix a bike at one in the morning, there are still greater moments for recreation and leisure in summertime.

But, did you know there is also a distinction between leisure and recreation? I bring this up because those who are instrumental in creating and organizing recreational programs for people with disabilities, more often than not, blend the two. Almost all of us blend the two. We think of fishing as leisure. In Canada, it is considered recreation by rehabilitation professionals. Walking or rolling outdoors in early evening with others, experiencing the day go down and night come up, is leisure. Playing a chess game is recreation. In leisure, often there is spontaneity, play, and laughter. Leisure time usually involves socialization. Obligations are few.

133

"Recreation is an activity taken up during leisure time. Leisure, on the other hand, is a 'state of mind;' a lifestyle; something that is entirely voluntary; something beyond the activity itself; something that gives life balance and meaning," authors Peggy Hutchison and Judith McGill state in their book, *Leisure, Integration, and Community* (Leisurability Publications, Canada, 1992).[1]

They go on to say, "[persons with disabilities] rarely have opportunities to go beyond enrollment in recreation programs or rarely have casual experiences in recreational activities, even when there is a interest [on their part] in doing so."

Why? Persons with disabilities often are segregated, bunched together, or isolated. This is partly due to inaccessibility, poor transportation, or an able-bodied person's fear of possibly becoming a disabled individual also. To leisurely walk with one who is disabled means looking squarely, and openly, at this person's disability. As you do so, your own fear(s) may crop up. Okay, now what? One thing is to become friends with your fears. Too, talk about that with your companion on the walk. As you probably know by now, I am a great proponent of communication. Talking about the unknown certainly dissipates any mystery, any fear.

One of my favorite leisure activities is, and always has been, taking a walk. Some of us need and use tools to get around, such as canes, crutches, wheelchairs, or motorized rickshaws. But there is no doubt about our ability to get out there. We just mainly need access. The outdoors has been a lifetime passion of mine, and that is partly why I walked so much. However, when I was walking in the past, I was often doing other recreational activities such as climbing, backpacking, or cross-country skiing. But whenever in Europe, I simply did more of the leisurely stuff. I just walked.

It's interesting to note that in Europe, almost every city with a lake or a river nearby has a well-used path running alongside. In fact, Geneva is famous for its paved paths running alongside the shore of Lac Leman. And most of these paths would end up somewhere, like the next town, village, or restaurant. These paths were a great way to visit my Geneva friends. And starting early in the morning, there also would be the exercisers, like fast-walkers, joggers, and ski-freaks on single-blade roller skates with ski poles for balance. Then came the commuters who rode their bikes to work. And if the weather was decent, the mothers with infants in strollers would appear.

Now, I can no longer walk. I use a motorized rickshaw for mobility. However, my love for the outdoors has not changed at all. I suspect this is true of many in the disability community. It's not that we don't care for taking a walk in the outdoors. It's just largely an inaccessible space. So, can you envision pathways suitable for wheels, designed with sensitivity to the environment and its natural inhabitants, and conducive to good mental and physical health for absolutely everyone?

Therapists, advocates, designers, family members, friends, and a host of others need to think about how to encourage the growth of leisure time and space for those with disabilities. Leisure can help to shape a person's identity, disabled or not, and change not only the perceptions others have of the person, but his or her own self-perception. How to encourage this? Persuade someone to strengthen an existing interest, or begin something entirely new with them. Do an art project together. Take a walk together. Go to the ball game together. But be spontaneous in doing so. Find other ways to bring persons with disabilities, big or little, into the fabric of community life, as big or as little as the occasion may be.

I would urge professionals such as architects or urban planners to create aesthetic, accessible plans that support the integration of leisurely or recreational activities for all. However, we must realize that community effort is needed as well. We can no longer usher persons with disabilities off to the professionals, to a dark corner, to a place away from our thoughts or activities. Remember, "they" can become "us" anytime. And would you want to be corralled off to some programmed activity instead of just casually meandering outdoors with a friend or two?

We need to start with personal introspection, to reflect on the right of all individuals to be part of our community. Also, we need to reform services. Services, which are highly organized and planned activities, and which become more recreational in nature than leisurely because of this very planning, are all that are available to many individuals with disabilities. Of course, such organized services can be partially ameliorated by any casual community support.

For any person with a disability, leisurely and spontaneous happenings can mean upgrading their personal life skills, adding confidence, and making them feel like a greater part of their community. For the general public, the interaction among all continues to educate about true integration, and about life beyond a wheelchair.

On Gardening

As a leisurely pursuit, let's look at gardening. Varied as plants are the reasons for a garden. It could be a full-fledged truck garden or a patch of lawn just big enough for a chair. We may be dilettantes or fanatics in our growing endeavors, and our pride in the results can be equally overgrown or sparing. Our gardens can have an impressionistic French-country look or the look of a pristine Japanese layout. Tiniest of seeds grow in ways so different that gardens are never the same, even if in the same place. But, a place it is.

When I was newly disabled, I wept and raged and grieved. Where I could do this most freely turned out to be in my garden space. The garden's ear turned to me. It listened and calmed me. This place accepted my rage and tears while continuing to quietly grow and give. Slowly, with the sprouting plants, my self-esteem grew back again—and grew with the acceptance of a new me. My garden helped the healing process tremendously. And it gave back to me a sense of leisure with its feeling of timelessness.

According to Diane Relf, assistant professor in the Department of Horticulture at Virginia Polytechnic Institute, Blackburg, Virginia, "Gardening is perhaps one of the oldest healing arts; yet as a science, it is very new among the thera-peutic professions." This new science is called horticultural therapy. Somewhat recreational in design, it can also become leisurely in activity.

The American Horticultural Therapy Association (AHTA)[2] describes itself as follows:

> Horticultural therapy involves the use of plants and plant related activities in improving the body, mind, and spirits of people. Through this approach to the therapeutic and rehabilitative treatment of people with special needs, horticul-ture has become a universally accepted and very effective tool in improving the quality of life of those whom the professional horticultural therapist serves.

Professional horticultural therapists work with individuals of all ages, including many who are experiencing some kind of disability. These therapists work in hospitals, correctional facilities, vocational training centers, alcohol and drug reha-bilitation centers, nursing homes, work co-ops, and a variety of other settings. Briefly, AHTA believes in self-medicating on horticulture. Horticultural therapy, in fact, is now taught in institutions of higher learning and has its own professional society, the aforementioned AHTA, and its own publications. It is considered a hands-on therapy.

True, plants have always played an important role in the physical and spiritual health of humankind. Trees were con-sidered divine in many ancient cultures; and today, herbs are still used for their medicinal properties. Equally, the wide-spread healing powers of gardening are not surprising. Some-one once said, "He is happiest who hath power to gather wisdom from a flower." And Isamu Noguchi furthered that with, "Nature is where we go to experience life."

According to *Newsweek's* predicted trends for the nineties, the watchword is, "If you want us, we'll be in the garden." Because of this, people are growing out into the community. Take the Tamarand Foundation, an organization that "creates green spaces for gardens and the arts within, on top of, or adjoining a dozen health-related facilities throughout the New York area." One of its cofounders, Bruce Detrick, says, "We work in the belief that life is nurtured by life; that the spirit may be whole though the body is ill. We have seen and are documenting the fact that the combination of music and nature offers a powerful complement to traditional medical and social services."

And, delightfully, you do not have to be disabled nor recovering from some illness to benefit from working in the garden. There are even gardening programs for healthy seniors. Look at the Gardening and Nutrition Project in Eugene, Oregon, which helps seniors feel less isolated and become more self-reliant. Because poor nutrition plays part of the solitary elderly lifestyle and because up to seventy percent of old peoples' physical ailments can be attributed to poor eating habits, this project takes a proactive role in promoting such activities. "Blending gardening with nutrition is the magical key," observes Robert Hackman, director of the project.

True, the garden is a place for so many of us, for so many reasons, and for endless benefits. And equally true, we all have needs. The garden should be one. As Lily Tomlin astutely observes, "For a quick fix, try slowing down." Plants will certainly do that to us.

But what do you do with a postage-size backyard of boring sorts? How do I design a garden that is accessible for me and my rickshaw and is easy to take care of as well? Yesterday, in the mail, comes the Seeds of Change[3] catalog, for organically-grown seeds, that plays havoc with my bank account. I dare not open it—yet. And with Plants of the Southwest being so close to where I live, I frequently pass by it when out on errands—so I look the other way to avoid temptation. Then my roommate, Karuna, comes home with a flier. Upon opening it, I see:

What Lives
in the Soul
Manifests
in the Garden;
What Lives
in the Garden
Grows
in the Soul.

Oh YES. This is it. This is what I am to think about right now. Nourishment. Nature. The soul. Not about problems. Not about the winter. Not about finishing this book. But about life. Yes. YES. YEESS.

With all the aforementioned, I realize there is something in the air—and in the soil. I respond. And act. I speak with one of the co-directors of the gardening organization whose flier I just received. One of their purposes is to help build gardens for people with disabilities. We make arrangements to get together tomorrow. Ideas just grow. Can I plant enough flowers to leave bouquets at nursing homes? Can I have an excess of vegetables to give to persons living with AIDS? All this is certainly worthy of thought instead of paying attention to the lousy weather outside.

Finally, the next day. Linda is here. We talk about all the above topics and then some. We talk about raised beds, the kinds that are just the right height and width for a wheelchair user. The concept excites me. Due to increasing balance problems and stretching limitations, gardening activities have slipped out of my life. With this, I can grow a garden once again. YES. I am excited.

Raised beds. They are rectangular, squares. I prefer circles. Round edges are softer. But in this case, I have no choice. So, why don't we follow the example of Chaco Canyon here in New Mexico, the straight paths leading to a center, the raised beds leading to a gazebo, much like spokes of a wagon wheel leading to its axle? Excitement mounts some more.

The day before the arrival of the spirited volunteers, who are largely from the Albuquerque region—actually, if you ask me, they are from heaven, bringing with them touches of the earth—a truckload of dirt comes. This black gold pile, a combination of organic sandy loam, compost, bark mulch, and manure, smells wonderful. Like the warm ground that you would lie on, the smells remind me of the days I would rest on the earth and watch the clouds while chewing on some dried plant stem. Fragrances bring back these wonderful memories, no?

Rain was forecasted for the next day, but everyone assembles regardless. Of course, the weather behaves. It is sunny and clear; a bank of clouds merely covers the nearby mountain peaks. We are in the sun, of course. That was part of the plan. After meeting one another and joking around, construction begins. The energy is high. Excitement swells. To have an accessible garden. Oh my. Yes, indeed!

The crew built and filled the beds in less than three hours. Co-director Linda hands me a prayer flag. On this white cloth flag is a transferred photo-image of a window at a meditation center. The window looks out at a garden, of course. We put the flag on the top of one of the arbor posts. Like a weather vane, it reveals a westerly wind. A storm is coming.

With the azure blue skies and now gathering puffy clouds overhead serving as a picturesque backdrop to this prayer flag, I feel wholesome, total, as I look at it. I do not feel my disability. I am delirious. Yes! And the heavenly soil is so very accessible, no longer out of my reach. I can now dirty my fingernails with black gold once again. How fashionable.

Later, as I plant the sugar peas, a friend, Michael, visits. I ask him if I am planting enough sugar peas to give away to people living with AIDS (PLAs). Michael has been working with PLAs for years. We talk about how it's the little things that mean a great deal for individuals contending with so much, sugar peas included. Then, I make a mental note to buy some statice seeds so I can bring colorful bouquets of dried flowers to nursing home residents as well.

Remember, it's the "practice random kindness and senseless acts of beauty" thing. Michael tells of gourmet restaurants in Santa Barbara, California, that give away their extra meals to PLAs. I tell Michael of my thwarted efforts to organize a similar growers group last year, of my frustration at not having enough energy to overcome these obstacles, at not being able to physically practice random kindness.

Well, energy is still low, but this year the obstacles shall not be a hindrance. First of all, I have an accessible garden. Second of all, it doesn't matter where you live or what kind of disability you may have. There is probably ground around you. Speaking about recreation, do re-create. And do be most leisurely about it.

On Libraries

A mother of a nine-year-old deaf child called to discuss the inaccessibility of our libraries. They are, very. And I am pained by it. Pained, because libraries have been a great source of leisure, among other things. Most of us, disabled or not, love books. Many persons with disabilities simply do not have enough discretionary income to buy books, so libraries do play an important role in our lives.

Thinking back, I have particular memories of two libraries. Growing up, I remember going often to our San Francisco neighborhood library with Dad. What a genuine place it was — and incredibly inaccessible as well. It was in a stately building one block north of Haight street and five blocks west of Ashbury street. I was walking then, and of course did not notice the steps leading up to the main entrance.

Years later, in 1989, I rolled into a relatively new library situated in a small town on the west coast of Sweden. Because there were no barriers for me and my wheelchair, I did not notice the effortlessness in getting around. I took that, like the steps in San Francisco, for granted. I did notice, however, just how much I enjoyed myself and just how much I felt part of the community, even if I could not read Swedish.

I want to go into great length describing this library because of its easy access to so much for so many. What a totally integrated, relaxed environment. From the very young to the old, from the able-bodied mother to her child with a disability, independence of use and movement was the mode. The ambiance of this three-story octagonal library embraced a completely relaxed culture. It was designed for leisurely pursuits.

On the ground floor in the center of the library's three-story atrium were big easy chairs, and of course, space for your wheelchair, to read whatever you had. Or simply to be. We were greeted by light-colored oak bookshelves under the big, circular balconies of this octagonal building. Visually, the place was very easy to see in because it was flooded with natural, indirect light. Next to the low, reachable stacks of books on the first floor, to maintain both the quiet and natural light, was a glass-partitioned playroom for kids. Since it was strategically located next to the checkout desk and visible from other viewing points throughout the library, adults could keep an eye on the kids. Or instead one could take the child along in a stroller complete with a book-carrying rack.

The third floor, where the newspaper racks stood, included a coffee shop and outdoor balcony overlooking the cobblestone streets and nearby port. Ever had good Swedish coffee and pastry at a library on an outdoor balcony in a wheelchair? That is what I call being leisurely at a premium.

Our director of libraries has a similar vision for the libraries here where I live. The details may not be exactly the same, but he does envision universal access for the very small, the big, the blind, the deaf, the young, the old, the physically able and not so able, and more. After all, they say, "What works for people with disabilities, works for many others as well."

For universal access to be successful, we must keep this in mind, always and in all ways. It is logic so well demonstrated in the small-town Swedish library described above. Many do envision the day when people can have complete access to the libraries via one's home computer. Such access is already happening via the Internet. In fact, we can probably visit this very Swedish library on the world wide web. But, flags of caution do arise. First, sitting at a home-based computer can be very isolating. And isolation is one of the biggest situations persons with disabilities face, let alone finding any money to buy a computer.

Second, in the zeal for creating accessible libraries, architects who follow building standards such as those set by the ADA (Americans with Disabilities Act) will find some of their provisions falling short of true accessibility for many people. Take for example the requirement that light switches be a maximum forty-eight inches above the floor. Architects tend to read that requirement to be exactly forty-eight inches high, and in they go, forty-eight inches up, meeting the requirements of the law.

But, for many, forty-eight inches is uncomfortably high. It is the *maximum* height suggested by ADA architectural guidelines, not the height most useful for many persons with disabilities. So life experience is best sought before final design is completed. It is certainly cheaper to change on paper than to do any costly retrofit in the building later on. And there is nothing more disruptive to a leisurely activity than having to struggle with something.

But to be fair, there should be no finger pointing, no addressing of single shortcomings. There are too many variables—everyone has different needs—and the ADA offers no panacea in this regard. What does this mean? It implies that an accessible, inclusive, humane society is the responsibility of *everyone,* absolutely everyone, from the architect to the zoo worker.

On a Recreational Activity

They call it freedom in the steep and deep. You know, skiing. I thought I'd attempt it, the Lovelace/Sandia Peak Ski Program for the Disabled offering me a try. Why not? After all, before rolling about in my motorized rickshaw, I skied a great deal, including bumming about on the slopes in Europe for two winters.

The person who inspired me to return to the slopes was Jimmie Heuga, a former Olympian who captured the bronze metal in slalom racing at the 1964 Winter Olympics in Innsbruck, Austria. But that was a long time ago. In fact, I barely remember it. Before I say anything about my current skiing affair, let me tell you what kind of medals Jimmie is now adding to his name. Pardon my putting him on another pedestal, as that is the last thing he now needs. But back in 1970, six years after the Innsbruck Olympics, he was diagnosed with multiple sclerosis (MS). Seven years later found him on the slopes again. That fact is certainly more valuable than a bronze medal.

What happened? Despite constraints imposed on him by the MS, Jimmie pulled himself out of a state of physical inactivity and worked on recapturing his health and fitness through a self-imposed, rigorous training program. He began bicycling over twelve hundred miles every year and swimming fifty laps per day, four times a week. He still does all that—and then some.

Of course Jimmie's previous athletic training helped. His accomplishment demonstrated to skeptics the validity of such exercise for people with MS, and he started a program based on his experiences, a program now known as the Jimmie Huega Center in Avon, Colorado, not far from Vail.

I ask Jimmie what skiing means to him today. He says, "The outdoors, namely the blue sky, mountains, forests, fresh air, wind and sun, have been an inspiration for me to reach my potential, for me to live my dreams." I think for many of us, able-bodied or not, in like manner, the outdoors feeds our dreams—and inspires. And so, I share my own experiences on Sandia Peak with you.

> January 16, 1991. I meet with Amy Cavanaugh, director of the Lovelace/Sandia Peak Ski Program. She is slight in build, pleasant in appearance, and enthusiastic in demeanor. We iron out last minute details. I ask her more. It turns out she is a Winter Park, Colorado, refugee. Winter Park has the oldest skiing program for the disabled in the United States. In fact, it began in 1969. Prior to working here, Amy had been there ten years.

> It is the day before the first lesson. I ponder my outfit. And in today's mail I find a surprise from someone. A Norwegian sweater. What a blessing, a positive omen.

Someone once said, "There is no such thing as an coincidence. It is God being anonymous." So I think this ski experience is to be good one — snow, pine trees, blue skies, and very fresh air. Oh Lord, do I need it. There is war. And the snow is white. White is the color of peace. The sweater's background color is also white.

The first day. It is the usual, friendly, outdoorsy ambiance at the base of Sandia's ski run. Lots of people. Lots of color. And very New Mexico blue skies. My instructors, Gary and Ernie, offer warm greetings and much help, help that is full of banter and free of the patronizing garbage.

You see all kinds of disabilities: amputees, muscular dystrophy, cerebral palsy, paraplegia, quadriplegia, and blindness to name a few. Not so visibly disabled, but equally very part of the program, are those with head injuries, the developmentally-disabled, the hearing-impaired, and the learning-disabled. All kinds. All ages. In other words, quite a crowd, and a happy one at that. It feels like carnival day up here. We enjoy the jostling, instructors included. They are stockbrokers, teachers, state employees, doctors, students, and you name it.

Gary and Ernie fit me into a sit ski. It is like a cross between a sled and a kayak. I feel inordinately clumsy, being towed and pushed up the beginners slope. We ski down maybe fifty feet a couple of times. Freedom in the steep and deep?

The following week. It is warmer today. Again, the sky is azure blue. I hope to get beyond the rudimentaries. I must unlearn everything I previously knew and must relearn this very new technique. I traverse less, turn more. There is a hint of freedom. Gary and Ernie offer encouragement. Not the "good girl" kind, but words of the sincere spirit that is shared among skiers. It is as refreshing as the mountain air. I try harder.

One instructor comments on the rush she gets watching the students improve. She says it is like doors to inner happiness opening up.

A week later, we take the chair to the top. The snow is packed powder up here. There are fewer people. With sit skiing, instead of the bend-the-knees rule, it is the wiggle-thy-hips. I do that more, and movement on the slope becomes easier. Things click. I face the fall line like a dancer before music. A mobility regained.

The runs are long, our breaths, short. We stop to inhale deeply and to take pictures. My eyes, despite the sunglasses, are watering from the rush. They are tears of freedom. I watch the chair lift overhead and the skiers below. It is a wonderful day. We shove off again to ski.

CHAPTER 14

ON TRAVEL, VACATIONS, NAPS, AND THEN SOME

Itching to see beyond your window, beyond the classroom, beyond the office, beyond any virtual-reality adventure, beyond, beyond—regardless of your limitation? Well, if you think the barriers are too great, there are some superb resources by and for people with disabilities regarding travel.

Before delving into a couple of these resources, let me share with you the excitement of traveling. Written in the early summer of 1989, here is a bit about my departure overseas for a three-and-a-half-month writing/photography grant project in Canada and Scandinavia, wheelchair included.

> With plane running down the runway, I get a rush, finally. The trip is on, the climb begins. I sink back into the seat and feel flashes of previous mountaineering trips I did before becoming disabled—the detailed, involved, and complex preparations; the checking and redundant rechecking; the lists and redundant lists; the looking over equipment; the counting ounces; the hassles. Oh

147

my Lord, this trip demands much of the same kind
work, but is a shade unlike any expedition in that I
wouldn't be halfway up a mountain to discover a missing piece of equipment.

The unknowns, however, felt as awesome, with my traveling overseas in a wheelchair for the first time. And
the strain of such intense preparations eclipsed any feelings of pre-departure excitement. So on the plane, I
just relished the solitude of the flight's first class plush-
ness, my being moved to that section for the entire leg
from Albuquerque to Toronto, Canada, for reasons unknown. Apparently, passengers in first class do not talk
to each other, and for once, I was glad . . .

Yet, regardless of all the reading, research, and planning
you may do, the unexpected invariably happens. As a friend
once said, "Nobody can predict a surprise." Prior to a five-day
visit to New York City I tried investigating just how accessible the city would be. Typical to New York style, there were
ten different replies to each specific inquiry.

I called those travel agents that claimed to specialize in
accessible travel. A mistake. Nine times out of ten, these agents
were able-bodied people that were unaware of an "accessible"
hotel's too-narrow bathroom door or the "little" four-inch
step down to the art gallery's main showroom. Their intentions may have been good, but they lacked the necessary experiential base.

Granted that travelers with disabilities need to be planners, and meticulous ones at that. But how about broken
wheelchairs, missing parts, an unexpected illness? How do
you plan for that? Fortunately, with the growing number of
persons with disabilities traveling — and why not? — resources
are equally growing. In a strange location, with a disability, in
trouble, and with a list of local Travelin' Talk[1] members on
hand, there can be help merely a phone call away. This is a
volunteer network of persons with disabilities, spread throughout the country and internationally. Members can call each
other for travel assistance. Because the information shared is

based on personal experience, it is accurate. A "little" step or narrow doorway is not overlooked.

Headquartered in Clarksville, Tennessee, Travelin' Talk was founded by a paralyzed veteran of the United States Air Force, Rick Crowder. The network currently spans North America from Anchorage to Miami and from Ottawa westward to Honolulu. There are members in over three hundred locations, including such international locations as Australia, Canada, China, India, Italy, New Zealand, Nigeria, Puerto Rico, South Africa, and West Malaysia. And Rick says, "We're growing larger by the day."

On to other traveling resources. Read *The Real Guide: Able to Travel* (1993, Prentice Hall/Travel, edited by Alison Walsh). Writings garnered from a hundred people with all kinds of disabilities, and from many places, reveal enough ventures to provide ample food for thought, if not outright action. Their stories are full of adventures ranging from good to bad, from Africa to Venice, and from living with cerebral palsy to being blind. In fact, the cover photograph of this guide book is of two elephants with passenger chairs riding on their backs, each carrying a man. Tied to the back of the large seats on top of the elephants are lightweight wheelchairs. The setting looks like Nepal or Northern India. Need I say more?

Despite the editor's choice not to substitute or delete language such as "confined to a wheelchair," "the halt," "the lame," "the infirm" or some questionable comments of the authors, such as "Santa Fe has an interesting range of architecture, mostly wheelchair accessible . . ." (a rather dubious claim if you ask me), the book is nevertheless a good read. In fact, it is so thorough and enjoyable that *anyone* might read it. For those thinking about an actual destination, if not an easier adventure than elephants in Nepal, the travel notes at the end of each section serve as a good jumping-off point for further research. Equally, the last chapter, on practicalities, is precisely that, practical. But for travelers with a disability, a great deal changes daily. Some of the stories, even dating back a couple of years, are no longer current. Fortunately, most of the changes have been for the better, due to both increased awareness of differing needs and the understanding that persons with disabilities spend their money just like any other tourist.

As Susan Sygall of Mobility International USA[2] says in the foreword of *The Real Guide,* "Perhaps it [the book] will encourage those who have only dreamed of travel, perhaps it will allow us to plan new adventures, and perhaps it will educate everyone that people with disabilities have a right to travel, to experience the unknown, the joys and disappointments, and the feeling that we are all part of a single planet that needs to bring its family closer together."

Back to the New York adventure. I wrote the following:

> Given any Sunday, any direction of the compass, wander. Something is happening. Everywhere. Being typical tourists, we headed for Central Park. With the main drive blocked off to weekend traffic, we joined all the other alternative, wheel-like locomotives that day. There were roller skaters, little to big, serious to whimsical. Bikes of all kinds wove asunder, including those umbrella carriage types built for, and often carrying, four riders at a time. And the horse-drawn buggies appeared with insistent regularity, followed by their diligent pooper scoopers, of course. I rolled by in a wheelchair, and viewed both Central Park and Manhattan from a navel-level, and then some, perspective.
>
> Meanwhile, there are over a million persons with disabilities in New York City (NYC) alone. I didn't see many. Now I understand why. Walking around Manhattan requires skill, agility, quick feet, and slim hips. The massive choreography and maneuver of pedestrians and vehicles alike somehow work. But wheelchairs—well, they don't have slim hips or quick feet. Maneuvering in such traffic can leave one a bit dazed. Yes, the curb cuts are there, but inconsistently so, and some with a three-inch drop.
>
> I did meet other New Yorkers in electric three-wheel scooters and wasted no time asking them to share with me their getting-about-NYC secrets. One person

carries her own sidewalk mini-ramp. Another simply drives on the street until the next appropriate curb cut. Heroic, I thought. But I'd rather close my eyes, hold my nose, and jump off a ninety-foot high dive into a tub of water. It seems easier.

Fortunately, there is more good help available. A resource that deals with sites well beyond NYC is a directory called *A World of Options for the Nineties: A Guide to International Educational Exchange, Community Service, and Travel for Persons with Disabilities*.[3] More than a packed directory, this guidebook also provides marvelous armchair traveling with personal stories ranging from a solar eclipse cruise in Southeast Asia to a study tour in London. Want to know the secrets of traveling on Amtrak with a wheelchair? Check out this detailed resource. Concerned about traveling with a specific disability? See the listing of disability-specific tours. Plus there are travel agents who can take you to any place on the face of the earth, travel agents with actual experience and understanding. By embracing the mottoes "Where there's a will, there's a way," and "Show yourself!" you feel very empowered by merely reading this guide.

Of another trip, I wrote:

> From the lush flatlands of Miami to the hills of San Francisco, I spent the holidays rolling about visiting friends and family. Pleasurable as these times were with others, traveling in a wheelchair was, ironically, not easy—for me or for anyone else who may have been involved in helping me.
>
> My childhood friend in Miami had ramps made so I could access their stair-laden home. Her husband chased all over town to rent a commode with grab bars. Numerous times throughout the visit, I was physically hauled in and out of the car. At the end of the stay, I am sure my dear friend was far more exhausted from all the efforts than I was. Then I headed for the other coast.
>
> Having grown up walking the streets of San Francisco, it was an eye-opener to revisit the place for the first

time in a wheelchair. My favorite columnist, Herb Caen, memorably refers to San Francisco as "last of the big splendors . . . a poor, beautiful, falling apart, torn-up San Francisco, loved one minute, reviled the next."

I agree in more ways than one. Not always able to get about in the inaccessible places, I was lifted, carried, and transferred. Thank goodness my brothers have decent backs. Others had the frightening experience of dropping me during a transfer. Fortunately, having been a long-time skier, I knew how to fall. So I was fine. But regardless, I love The City, having been born there. It is home. Inaccessible as it may be.

The cabbies there, however, are no different than those worldwide. Coming back from an office visit, the cab driver found himself dislodging me from a tight squeeze between his car door and a sidewalk tree, the result of his careless parking. As my brother sarcastically commented later, "After all, these guys have a reputation to maintain." More laughter.

I also made the mistake of assuming that the home of one of my relatives was accessible, as it was claimed. I failed to take my own advice: never ask an able-bodied person about accessibility. Such erroneous information continued during our efforts to find a hotel room with accessible features for the second half of my stay. Moral: Despite the increasing awareness and good intentions of others, persons with disabilities need to prepare by contacting other persons with disabilities and sticking with information and resources offered from the disability community only, such as the aforementioned Travelin' Talk network.

I had no idea what it would be like returning home after three strenuous weeks traveling from coast to coast. During my time away, mobility limitations were severely felt. Lo and behold, I arrived at my small, adobe home in Albuquerque to discover something joyous. Being accessible in every way, it was so easy to move about, to do things in this house. The lift-equipped, hand-controlled van outside proved equally liberating. Instead of exhaustion, I felt emancipated.

Nevertheless, the topic of travel is always germane for most of us anytime, disabled or not. Of my latest vacation, I wrote the following:

> Dog days are here. I am into the summer routine. Work permits me to take a siesta between two and four in the afternoon, after putting in a long morning of writing. Around 4 P.M., I wake up to frozen yogurt, continue to cool off while checking the news, then spend time outside, among the garden, neighbors, and by this time, among the now active dogs, cats and kids. After dinner and more phone calls, I return to writing.
>
> The summer days are slow like that, slower in many respects. Vacation or no vacation, I am now getting to love this slower season. As E. B. White so beautifully writes — which must be shared with you — he captures the essence of these hot summer days:

> At eight of a hot morning, the cicada speaks his first piece. He says of the world: heat. At eleven of the same day, still singing, he has not changed his note but has enlarged his theme. He says of the morning: love. In the sultry middle of the afternoon, when the sadness of love and of heat has shaken him, his symphonic soul goes into the great movement and he says: death. But the thing isn't over. After supper he weaves heat, love, death into a final stanza, subtler and less brassy than others. He has one last heroic monosyllable at his command. Life, he says, reminiscing. Life.

I read something by Barry Corbet, writer, outdoors man, disability advocate, and editor of *New Mobility*[4] magazine, that got me reflecting. What is so lamentable about his remark is its truthfulness. Corbet refers to the fact that the disabled never get a vacation.

Why? Our disability follows us like a shadow. It is always there, always, in all ways. Our shadow of disability(s) is even there on a rainy day. The struggle of daily survival for any person with a disability is perpetual and unrelenting, no matter what the disability, no matter the locale. Even for the able-bodied individual on vacation, being in an unfamiliar environment is a trying task. So for a person with a disability, taking a shower or dining away from home in unpredictable circumstances becomes an awesome chore, taking away much of the fun of the vacation. Consequently, for a person with a disability, it is very difficult to fall into a totally relaxed mode on vacation.

But I have had a wonderful vacation, albeit short, far too short. It was right here at home. My younger brother came down from San Francisco for a brief visit. During his stay, during the heat wave, he drove me around, washed the living room rug, set up my new VCR, tightened kitchen cabinet hinges and more. With the exception of the driving, I never asked for anything. How utterly relaxing his visit . . .

We visited friends, ate well, watched the Wimbledon, and made a surprise group call with others on my speaker phone to a dear old crony in Switzerland. We laughed a lot, exchanged thoughts, talked about the family, about disability issues, checked out a secondhand store, gossiped with neighbors, and even took naps. Because my brother essentially made life easy for me during his stay, I had a vacation, a wonderful break from the daily efforts of life and felt very rested after his visit.

On the subject of naps, the other day I forgot to put the phone on the answering machine and was awakened from an afternoon siesta with a ringing phone. The caller was somewhat concerned after my saying "Good afternoon," with a voice fuzzy from sleep. When I explained that I just awakened from a long nap, she said, "What a luxury!" For some of us, it is. For others, an absolute necessity. Naps are minivacations. In the rest, I travel. Essentially, I escape my disability for two hours while taking a trip into the subconscious, a fascinating place. Naps are what you can call restful traveling and immense restoration.

If you know someone with a disability, know that a vacation for a person with a disability can occur right at home with your help, especially if naps are included. The key is being aware of their needs and then taking an initiative in doing the necessary. Though architect Mies van der Rohe was referring to designing buildings when he said, "God is in the details," this line also applies to people, especially in the aforementioned situation. In other words, be sensitive, be aware of the surrounding needs. Then be appropriately proactive. Attend to details. Give a vacation. Give a break.

And for the person with a disability, with luck you can relax, giving slack to any demand. Trust that this person knows. Just be. Enjoy the visit. Slow down. It's vacation time. And for both, have some fun.

CHAPTER

15

ATTENDANT CARE

Some of America's most cherished ideals include independence, individualism, and autonomy. So ingrained is this philosophy that it's evident in our very way of being, of thinking, and of everyday action. People with disabilities feel and think no differently.

Autonomy, self-control, and freedom also provide *everyone* a sense of well-being. However, there is an immense battle going on regarding this independence so dear to all of us. People with disabilities, and many elderly persons as well, are struggling at some point in their lives to live out this very basic tenet until their dying day. One possibility in dealing with this challenge is to hire at-home attendant care when needed.

Attendant care? "Hard to get." "Can't afford it." "I'm doing fine, thank you." "How does this piece of puzzle fit into my picture anyway?" "Besides, where do I find such a person?" "And what about things like trustworthiness?"

Interestingly, these questions loom for all of us, one time or another after diagnosis or injury. And as for me, my stubbornness and pride prevented me from seeing the light a few years. Not until living alone and after exhausting myself doing ordinary daily living activities (DLA), did I look at the possibility of hiring help on a regular basis. In doing so, I saved myself continued misery. It might even save your primary relationship. Obviously, a partner, though not subject to the vagaries of the disability itself, is unquestionably very affected by the impact the disability can have on all of us.

So a different way of looking at this is that you are not only hiring attendant help for yourself, but are easing up the situation for all those around you. Hiring attendant care actually *adds* to the value of your relationship with others. It is saying, "I love you. I care about you. And I care about us." You don't have to be married for this to happen. You could be saying this to your parents, your siblings, your children, your partner, your roommate, or even to yourself. The central point here? Look at hiring attendant help for reasons quite different than you initially may have thought.

Let it be foresight, not hindsight. Permit yourself to accept the need. It is the act of kindness for all those you love and those who love you.

You are probably asking yourself, "How am I suppose to hire someone if I don't have any money?" For a long time, it was a familiar obstacle for me, mainly because I didn't know how to even begin with the logistics, including the basics such as who, when, why, for how long, and for how much. Where do I even go for advice?

You've probably heard the saying, "To learn what is down the road, ask those coming back." In America, we members of the disability community are incredibly blessed by the ever-sprouting centers for independent living (CIL) across the country. Run by and for people with disabilities, CILs associate independent living with attendant care services. Fortunately, local chapters of any organization intended to help persons with disabilities are making the connections as well. Simply, to reiterate, attendant care means independent living.

But back to the rudimentary: money. We need to learn how to ask—ask those who love us, our families, our churches.

If you explain how you plan to use the contribution, more folks than not will be pleased, very. Sometimes it is simply easier for them to dole out the bucks than do anything else. Too, it may alleviate any guilt on their part.

You hate asking? Then ask someone to ask for you. Better yet, give them a copy of this, then talk. Shy about talking? Then, contact one of the aforementioned centers to get connected to a recommended peer counselor. In so doing, you are asking someone who has been down the road. And learning how to ask for help . . .

Shy about associating with the disability community? It's okay. I was, too. In fact, it took me a long time to make the transition from one community to another. But the old axiom, "There is power in numbers," holds utterly true here.

You will find many of your old able-bodied friends falling away, not because of you, but because of the disability. Just as you were, your friends probably are scared. There is not much you can do about that. Face it, we are not a nation of very brave folks. However, you will be pleased to find that many members in the disability community not only bear purple hearts for their nonmilitary actions, but also are not afraid of your condition. In fact, you will be welcomed as you are, probably without any questions asked.

So now you have the money. How do you find the help? Remember, always ask those who have been down the road first. Usually, most any CIL will have a pool of names for you. If not, find a source that will help you with running a classified ad. Do not list your name, address, or phone number in the ad. This is where your source helps. Use their phone number and let them do the prescreening for you. Also, make it very clear that you will require references and will do background checks. The initial interview should be done at a place other than where you live.

Why the above precautions? Safety. One statistic after another reveals that people with disabilities, when abused, are often abused by the very person on which they are dependent, hired attendant help being no exception.

Then, if you follow the above guidelines well, there is the danger that you both will become friends. Danger? Well, the working relationship changes. To maintain the working relationship and the emerging friendship, you both need to be sensitive, aware, and adroit. In itself, this is a challenge.

So what to do with hired help? Before hiring anyone, record, or have someone record for you, the DLAs you find most tiresome, laborious, or frustrating to do. With this list, talk to your potential attendant about that, about both of your weaknesses and strengths, likes and dislikes. Within these parameters, write down a plan. Even though you are the boss, you discover a great deal about each other when making plans together. Plus, this person is putting into written words what he or she can, and will, do. This, in itself, can be a powerful commitment.

If this person is an experienced attendant, be open to suggestions. Proceed slowly. Discover what works well for both of you. Understand that one person cannot do everything. If you need to, hire a second or third person. The variety helps. Wisely, I leave the housecleaning chores with the housecleaning ladies. It is their specialty, they do it well, my attendants are relieved, and we're all that much more content.

A while back, I wrote the following story about what attendant care at home has meant to me.

> I weep. I weep tears of overwhelming gratitude, tears of immense relief, tears of utter weariness, and tears of pain over what my disabled brothers and sisters continue to endure.
>
> Easter Sunday my family calls to say they are helping. A check is on its way in the mail. I can now hire extra help. Someone can come in every day for a couple of hours. Whew. What a relief.
>
> My friend, Karuna, astutely remarks, "Karen, doing the everyday stuff is wearing you out. In fact, it's killing you." I now allow myself to see that. And I now realize the system is failing me, failing us, failing miserably.

I am tired. With reason. To do what might take a nondisabled person five-easy minutes takes me twenty-hard minutes, mildly stated. But, please understand, I am not complaining. It is simply a fact.

I say to others, "It's easier to write an article than clear the table." A sad, but true, anecdote. Life has been clouded by the endless, but simple, efforts. Even to brush my teeth involves imposing exertion.

Today, after work, I realize I can afford to relax. ReLAX. I forgot the meaning of that word. I roll the expression around my tongue as we do when tasting something new. Still, there are tears. But the struggles are to ease up, are easing up. Not that someone will brush my teeth, but, at least, I can rest after doing so.

Inhale, exhale, I tell myself. Learning to graciously accept so much help has been a new experience for me. I am touched. I cry. I am simply overwhelmed.

I was talking to friend, Avis, about my threshold of resistance in asking for any kind of assistance. The hesitancy comes largely from having to fare on my own for so long.

Avis responded by saying, "Karen, your family has probably always wanted to help, but didn't know how. It's a win-win situation now." But, of course. In hindsight, it hasn't been easy. And I still go through minor gymnastics asking for help. I simply did, and probably will continue to do, what had, has, to be done.

But now, instead of putting all my energy into simple survival, I can be freer to do the things I really want, things beyond the ordinary daily living activities. Just think, I will now have more energy to spend on deeds like writing about various other matters, pursuing my spiritual inclinations, carrying on with activist and community responsibilities, gardening, helping others, and just plain ol' relaxing with friends and children.

But the tears. They continue to flow. They are tears of gratitude and tears of frustration. And my scowl does not wash away. My family is not wealthy, not by any means. In ways, my struggle becomes their struggle, trying to make financial ends meet.

I frown because Medicare will easily pay up to $37,000 per year to house me in a nursing home, but it will not pay a cent toward hiring the help of my preference to come in for a couple of hours of assistance each day. Needless to say, hiring my own help is a great deal cheaper than $37,000 per year. Plus I am happier. I am in my own environment, doing what I want when I want. And my spirit is very nourished because of this, because of my garden, my pets, my adobe walls, and because of my own mess.

Why this? Well, the American Health Care Association (AHCA), with very, very deep pockets, operates the majority of nursing homes on a for-profit basis, and has one of the wealthiest and strongest lobbying organizations in the United States, if not the world.

In fact, according to the January 1995 issue of the *Provider*, the nursing-home industry trade magazine, the top ten nursing home chains increased their revenues by twenty-five percent in the last year. And they did this with no change in the number of beds. How's that? Well, to keep their reported combined income up, totaling some $9.2 billion last year, to keep their profits high, and to keep their lobbying organization healthy, AHCA hires cheap, if not unskilled, labor and literally "warehouses" their occupants for maximum efficiency and minimum effort.

No surprise. This downsizing of expenses is commonly practiced today by most big businesses. I cry some more. I sob for those who endure and suffer, for those who simply cannot afford it. They are the true victims. Many of my disabled brothers and sisters do not have a family that can help. So they struggle until no longer able to do so. Then, Medicare/Medicaid pays for their nursing home expenses. Often young, and in an alien environment, they wither away and die quietly.

It's time to start singing, "Where have all the wheelies gone? Long time rolling . . ."

It's a phenomenal waste of money, a waste of unnecessary taxes, a killing of spirit and then some, a financial drain for many, including my family, and loss of life uncalled for. I weep more. But also, they are tears of gratitude. Thank you family. I am spared.

Care seems to be a mixed experience for many of us. One definition in the *Webster's International Dictionary* says, "A burdensome sense of responsibility; trouble caused by onerous duties; anxiety; concern." Many of you involved in the "caregiving" or the "caretaking" of someone probably could not agree more with the above definition. But, Rev. Wayne Muller of Santa Fe, New Mexico, could not disagree more.

Before talking about Rev. Muller's thoughts on care, I'd like briefly to mention two issues surrounding care: namely, the needs of those providing care, any kind, and at anytime, and the needs of members within the disability community. In one way or another, we are all involved in care. It starts at a very early age, for example, with pet hamsters. Then we have younger siblings. This eventually evolves into raising our own kids. Add on assisting any temporarily injured or infirm individual. They, too, are "taken care of." There are also caregivers/caretakers or care providers that are involved in the welfare of their parents, those involved in the illnesses or injuries of their loved ones, those working in hospitals, in nursing homes, and within the disability community. Care is not only pervasive, but ongoing, and a constant thread that weaves throughout our lives.

Back to Wayne Muller. He is an ordained United Church of Christ minister and founder of Bread for the Journey, a grassroots community foundation in northern New Mexico. He is also a psychotherapist, pastoral counselor, husband, father, and more. Furthermore, Rev. Muller works with the AIDS Wellness Program team at the Visiting Nurse Service. In short, he is quite qualified to talk about care — and for the benefit of you "caregivers," I quote his thoughts on giving care. He has a marvelous perspective.

> Part of our voice as pastoral counselors is to question whether "care" is something we really "give" at all. Are we truly the source of all care? . . . When we call ourselves care "givers," that implies we must be the ones who "have" all the care to give. Like some secret stash, every moment we have to decide who gets it, and when, and how we parcel it out to those in need when the time comes. And then we have to find some way to "get" some more . . .

Along with asking astute questions about "caregiving/care-taking," Wayne Muller equally provides some answers.

> . . . What if care is something that gently waters the earth, something from which we all may drink, something that is infused in every mo-ment, if we will but hold one another, and listen, and remember? Perhaps we do not "give" care at all, but only remind one another to drink from the fountain of care to which we all are invited by the loving spirit of the earth. We need to remind ourselves that there is more than enough care to go around. We may find care in the color of the sky, a touch, the smell of a lilac, the feel of the earth as it presses against our feet, welcom-ing us as we walk.

Now, about those in need of assistance. It has become a vital issue. I cannot do much without my help now, and am, in an ironic sense, dependent on the very help that keeps me independent. Independent of what? Of institutional care. That is the nightmare of everyone, so much so that there are even articles now out about "How I escaped a nursing home."

Our society is used to calling the care I have been discuss-ing, "nursing care." We in the disability community call it "attendant services." It is more appropriate. There is nothing medical at all about the attendant services we receive. Yes, the AHCA would like care to fall under the auspices of "nursing" or "medical" care for apparent reasons. Having someone help you get up in the morning or do the laundry is obviously not nursing care. Common sense also will tell you that assistance with daily living activities such as eating, brushing your hair, or sweeping the floor does not require a nursing degree. Though nursing homes hire low-wage-earning individuals to do such, these institutions bill Medicare/Medicaid exorbitant fees for their "nursing" services. Such a loophole is costing the taxpayer untold, unnecessary dollars.

Denmark realizes that nursing homes create quagmires of emotional, financial, and other unpleasant sorts. In fact, Denmark is almost through phasing them out. Their solution? Fostering independence by a nationally-supported, in-home attendant service program. Interestingly, as I write this, there are movements here pushing for, and very close to realizing, change in this regard. Hopefully, by the time you are reading this, some of these changes will have taken place.

Going about hiring and managing at-home attendant care is one of the most proactive, sensible, and positive things you can do for yourself and your loved ones. As they say, "Make it happen."

CHAPTER

16

AGING

This is a difficult subject to approach because so little is known, or even acknowledged, about aging with a disability. We have always accepted the notion that as you get older, you become more disabled. As the saying goes, "People age into disability." It is a familiar marriage and pattern. Graying. Falls. Wheelchairs. Nursing homes — or does it have to be?

Too, we have bought into the notion, particularly here in America, of being forever young. In other words, you don't get older; you just disappear. But, aging with a disability? That marriage is not thought of, at least not very much, anyway.

As part of buying into the forever-young-syndrome, wheelchair users buy, and work out in, lighter and lighter manual chairs, hoping their added strength will carry them further. And within the disability community, to go from a manual wheelchair to a power wheelchair is thought of as giving in to your frailty. There is also the lose-what-you-don't-use fear. Does it have to be?

Then, there is the seemingly unrelated post-polio syndrome (PPS). More than forty years after getting polio, the survivors are now seeing a surge of the post-polio syndrome, or what also is called post-polio sequelae, in their ranks. The explanation for PPS suddenly occurring so many years later remains as mysterious today as when the symptoms of extreme fatigue, pain, and weakness first started appearing a few years back. But, as Patti Strong, a polio survivor and expert on aging with a disability, says, "Whereas it formerly was not understood that major damage could be present without paralysis (or even debilitating weakness), it is now known that muscles of only fifty percent strength can function apparently normally for about thirty years before an irreversible overuse weakness even becomes noticeable."

Though I don't have polio, the same aforementioned symptoms have plagued me, especially after a long, hot summer. Then, chair notwithstanding, I'd fall. A lot. So more effort. More blows. More weakness. More pain. And then, more effort. A truly vicious circle. Does it have to be? The truth is that with energy ebbing, I was simply trying to muscle my way through getting older. No wonder they say, "Pushing fifty is hard exercise."

Face it: I'm wearing out. So, too, I suspect—along with many others—are all the survivors now dealing with PPS. President Roosevelt had a point when he said that after spending two years trying to wiggle his big toe, being president was not that hard. In March 1996, *New Mobility*[1] magazine devoted an issue to polio. It also has a short, but fascinating, article on Tom Houston, a paraplegic after a construction accident in 1980, who is now fifty-five and planning to go, at least, another thirty years. And why not? Of course his diatribe is one about the combined stress and aging dilemma we all face. Of using manual wheelchairs and then some, Tom says,

> It's harder to wheel. It's harder to transfer and it's harder to dress, simply because I've used my arms in a mode they weren't designed for. I'd like to be able to dress and transfer myself in another thirty or forty years. I'm not going to be able to do that if my arms are totally worn out at age fifty-five.

When asked why any paraplegic in his right mind would want a power wheelchair, Tom fired back, "Why do able-bodied people drive automobiles? They don't ride bicycles, they drive automobiles." He goes on to say,

> We [persons with disabilities] need to look at tools that will help us get through a full day from morning to night and be productive, functional, and independent. And a manual chair doesn't really do that. It's very limiting. It's very energy-consuming. That's what powered mobility is about.

Tom has a point. When parts in our car wear out—and do they ever, so predictably so—we either replace them or, eventually, given the money, buy a new car. But, for someone like myself, replacing a worn-out part, usually via surgery, is a no-no, surgery being as damaging as the worn-out part itself. Buy a new body? In my next lifetime . . .

And, of course, taking all into consideration, there is a necessary balance. Regardless of age, a modicum of exercise is needed for our well-being. Moderation is the key. Too, diet is a consideration. After all, our stomach and heart are parts vulnerable to wearing out as well. Using tools such as power chairs to help us as we age is not a giving-in, but is an exercise in sensibility, a practical paradigm with which we should accept change gracefully.

Interestingly, the National Spinal Cord Injury Association,[2] in the Summer, 1995, issue of their magazine, *SCI Life,* has an article on aging titled, "Aging Bodies . . . Changing Needs," where individuals talk about wearing out, more bluntly referred to as aging, and in this specific case, aging with a disability. The comment, "It's all hindsight," echoes loudly in the words of these individuals. One says, "If I had treated my shoulders better when I was twenty, they'd probably be treating me lots better now that I am forty."

Before switching to a power chair, one person was worried about his fitness and muscles atrophying. The hindsight? He now says, "I have more energy, am more active, and [am] less

dependent." I, too, had the same fears of what would happen
if I relied on my motorized rickshaw more. But so far, so
good. After eight years of not walking, my leg muscle tone is
holding—it must be the modicum of exercise. After six
months of relying more on attendants, I have more energy
than I've had in years—it must be their help.

Good occupational and physical therapists can separate
simple aging factors from the emotional elements that can go
with disability, and can recommend changes in equipment or
the environment to meet the added needs of aging. As listed
in *SCI Life*, such recommendations usually are in response to:

- Lower strength and function

- Increased pain

- Decreased mobility

- Weight gain or loss

- Less activity

- Skin sores

- Posture problems

- Aging of the primary caregivers

As Patti Strong says,

> The most critical thing for professionals in
> aging to learn about aging with disability is [it's]
> new to everyone. Chronic disabling conditions
> [such as polio, MS, MD, chronic fatigue syn-
> drome] are not static. People with disabilities
> incur a double whammy to their independence
> as they age. Not only are we subject to the usual
> illnesses or weaknesses associated with aging,
> but our disabling conditions also change.

Sound familiar? Enough of the stoic. Enough worrying
about appearance, or what may be a perceived image, or dependency. Is not energy more important so you can continue
to be a good parent, do your job well, advocate lots, write a
book? And what about aging gracefully, disabled or not?

17

DIET, EXERCISE, AND HEALTH

Diet

For almost everyone, the holidays are the season of weight gain. For polar bears, weight gain in winter is not only acceptable, it's imperative. But for anyone else carrying excess weight, I need not explain in depth the connections to arterial disease, hypertension, stroke, diabetes, cancer, and more. For those of us with mobility problems, weight gain also can be risky because of such added complications as injury from a fall.

Transferring from a wheelchair to a car requires agility. Walking with any kind of assistance requires balance. A broken elbow from a fall may not seem like such a big deal, but for a person who has paraplegia of the legs, arms are vital. Too, for the more sedentary, additional weight slows down any kind of healing process. So, in more ways than one, staying slim plays a critical role for persons with disabilities.

A healthy diet, needless to say, is a healthy move on everyone's part, regardless of mobility status. More and more people realize this. In fact, a *USA Today* survey pointed out that two out of three people feel diet is more important than exercise in living a healthier life. That the average annual consumption of red meat is going down yearly, according to a late edition of the Census Bureau's *Statistical Abstract of the U.S.*, is an indication of such thinking.

Because of my condition, I've been on a low-fat diet for years. Recently, I needed to gain weight, and found it quite a challenge considering my dietary guidelines. It took me almost a year to gain twenty pounds since I did not want to depart from my low-fat patterns of eating. So successful is this low-fat diet that I'd like to share a little with you in the hope that my experience of staying slim might be useful.

One thing I've discovered in my concern for what I eat is the abundant lack of knowledge out there about fats. For example, take my favorite TCBY frozen yogurt place. When asked specifically for a nonfat selection, the vendors would often respond, "This one is sugar-free." Granted, sugar can make you fatter, but it is not the same thing as eating saturated fat. In ways, the ingestion of saturated fats is a lot worse than too much sugar.

A low-fat diet means largely eliminating saturated fats from your diet. Since saturated fats mostly come from animal products, that means knocking off the red meats and dairy products. They are real culprits. I have not eaten cheese in a long time. The skinned white meat of chicken or turkey is fine.

Dairy products. Fortunately, many products with one and a half percent fat contents are available, delighting the Stanford Heart Institute and myself. You can also get soy cheese substitutes at your local health food store. Some take getting used to, but have you tried the soy parmesan cheese? Friends say they cannot taste the difference.

Alcohol. Don't drink it. Coffee? Don't drink it either. Like any caffeinated product, it actually stimulates your appetite. Thus, the marriage between coffee and donuts is not such a coincidence. Energy level? The longer you abstain from such stimulants or downers like alcohol, the more vital your energy becomes. For example, yesterday afternoon, I ate half of a health food candy bar, and the little caffeine that it contained kept me up until two this morning. I need not tell you how spry I feel today.

Labels. Read them, but know that they're insidious. "Vegetable oils" do not necessarily mean fat-free. Your tropical oils such as coconut and palm actually promote weight-gaining. "Hydrogenated," even partially, should really read "saturated oil," again a no-no for those so concerned.

The list of pointers could be endless. You are probably confused and concerned. Granted, there is much more to say and more to learn. Educate yourself. The know-how of eating well is not handed out freely on a silver platter. Learn about good eating. Read classics such as *Laurel's Kitchen,* especially the introduction, for fine pointers in nutrition. Read Dr. Swank's book, *The Multiple Sclerosis Diet Book,* for the best explanation of fats and oils I've seen to date. You don't have to have MS to reap benefits from studying this. Have fun with the exotic, but healthy ways of eating found in the Moosewood cookbooks. And all of the above books contain wonderful recipes.

Low-fat or nonfat, I am eating very well, thank you. Simply, I try to eat wisely, always and at all times. Though I love polar bears, such chubbiness is certainly not needed here.

Exercise

Pull. Exhale. Release. Inhale. Feel the muscles. Feel the tension. Relax. And repeat. Three sets, ten times each. I work hard. But the slow going is a reminder that progress really is measured in centimeters, not miles.

Disability and exercise? You bet. The credo that disability is not synonymous with inability is so true here. We do what we can do, however we can do it. In the era of healthier lifestyles, exercise, along with the spiritual, loving, working, and growing parts of our selves, is considered vital. This physical activity is essential to the maintenance of our well-being, regardless of physical status. "Many persons with disabilities can slow down or stop any debilitating process . . . and the physical and psychological benefits have been well documented," says an instructor at the University of New Mexico's Therapeutic Physical Education Lab.

Another exercise place worth mentioning is the Jimmie Huega Center.[1] It's an organization that emphasizes exercise as a way to reanimate our life. The center evolved from the experiences of Jimmie Huega, one of the U.S. Ski Team's top racers for ten years. Conventional wisdom at the time of his diagnosis with MS dictated that he avoid physical exertion. He complied, but not for long. Previously being such a physically active person, he felt the sedentary approach was wrong. It left him feeling unhealthy, unmotivated, and tired. He came to several conclusions:

> I realized that MS had become my excuse to
> lose my physical health, and even more, to
> experience anxiety over becoming inactive. I
> decided that no matter where MS was going to
> take me, I was going to go in as good physical
> shape as I could. In other words, I decided that
> the most important characteristic of my life was
> the quality of each day.

So Jimmie began to ride a bike. This was not easy because of his poor balance. He fell a lot, but persisted. And a very strange thing happened to him:

> I experienced an exhilarating feeling which left
> me physically tired rather than mentally drowsy.
> It was like a nibble of the mainstream of life
> that had been passing me by and it was this
> modest program that really began to become
> self-reinforcing, and that changed the attitude
> that I had allowed myself to develop.

Because of his program's immense benefits, Jimmie Huega subsequently created a center espousing a healthier lifestyle for those with MS. There, exercise is a big component. He reminds us of a few points that actually are applicable to everyone:

- You have nothing to prove to anyone, so do it for yourself.

- You only have to live up to your own expectations, so put yourself first. Make time for your exercise programs and be selfish about your health.

- Set realistic goals based on your priorities, goals that are "do-able."

- By setting realistic goals, we have the opportunity to reclaim our self-confidence. This leads to a new feeling of self-esteem, and the outgrowth of accomplishments generate a renewed self image.

One of the best places for those with disabilities to exercise is in a pool. Water is considered a great equalizer among all. Even football players utilize aquatherapy to recover from injuries. The healthy 49ers take this a step further and use pools for conditioning.

Health

My journal says about a recent day,

> Up at 7:15 A.M. Through the usual routine and it's now 12:30 P.M. Am feeling exhausted plus some. Am finally writing, but where has all the time gone?

For persons with disabilities, we need not ponder long for an answer. The time is consumed doing ordinary, daily tasks. For those folks not dealing with any disability, it's hard to believe. These things are so taken for granted.

But in addition to daily activities, I am paying homage to the body, minding the temple so to speak. As usual, as soon as I felt better from a recent bout of illness, I started doing things again. Much too soon, much too quickly. A mistake.

So I paid dearly for it. Now, I am beginning to realize this is a lesson for me. I need to learn to go slowly, very slowly. I need to learn how to say, "No." Though the emotional and spiritual realms feel strong, my physical state is not—yet.

The saying, "First ecstasy, then laundry," makes much sense. Not that being ill was ecstatic—far from it—but working on a pile of laundry is certainly in the picture now. It seems that a balance should be created between the physical, emotional, and spiritual dimensions in our lives. Disablement? A fourth dimension, so it feels. So there is a great skill to be learned in the weaving of these dimensions which play an enormous factor in our well-being.

There is no formula for doing this. It is the dance of life. It is the spider making all the connections on the web hold. Some strands are shorter, some longer, but the idea of a web is to catch nourishment. The hope is for people, disabled or not, to learn to expand their web as well so as to encompass and nourish others. What does that mean? In part, I think, it is to honor each dimension—being as healthy, emotionally and physically, as possible, and being spiritually connected. For persons with disabilities, the added dimension of disablement means acknowledging, accepting, and living beyond the limits. It does not mean being a "Super Crip" or the "Exemplary Martyr." It means, in spite of it all, being human, being realistic. Like they say, "Be the best you can be." But be human, regardless.

During one of Albuquerque's earlier "Disability Awareness Weeks," I addressed students with disabilities at the University of New Mexico campus by saying the following:

> You are sharing so much with others this week, every day, on graduation, every moment. And you unwittingly are doing more. You are blazing trails . . . and becoming mentors to those coming after you. You are creating disability pride, disability cool. You are making this community visible and adding to the growth of our culture as a whole. You are showing others what it means to be human.

Back to the physical dimension: recently I have learned of new limits (they are always changing). And I owe it to myself and others to regain my health. I owe it to all those who have helped out, physically, in consideration, and in prayer. So now I go slow, real slow. And am doing very well in the turtle marathon, thank you.

18

ON THE JOB

With passage of the Americans with Disabilities Act, of course, we will see more and more persons with disabilities at work. Too, because of the shrinking work force, we are going to need everyone we can get on the job. According to numerous polls, the vast majority of unemployed persons with disabilities *want* to work. With these changes, working able-bodied persons will have questions concerning accommodations, behavior, teamwork, and mere coexistence. Likewise, persons with disabilities will have similar concerns. Addressing all here is not possible, but the ensuing story about my own work experience may offer some insight.

Previous to my disability, I worked as marketing coordinator for a large architectural-engineering firm. The process I went through for incorporating my disability into the workaday world seems to be of value to all of us.

After climbing mountains, walking with a cane, I thought, was a formidable enough challenge—let alone rolling about in a wheelchair. But little did I know of the challenges still waiting to be addressed, like communication. How do you convey a shaky day without shaking up your boss? How do you instill confidence, among coworkers, that you are still part of your playing team? How do you talk to people about your disability without scaring them off?

I thought, in my nondisabled days, that I was a sensitive enough person. The ability to listen and to understand friends, coworkers, and contacts, I practiced. I got that from Dad. He was a real heart-listener, one of those people who put himself in your shoes. If you were sitting in the gutter, he sat there alongside, simple as that. Needless to say, I thought these things were naturally passed on. Well, now disabled, I discovered that the most sensitive person in the world still cannot come anywhere near comprehending disability, not even a person like Dad. The ability to understand is not naturally passed on to the next generation. Each acquires it over time and mostly through experience.

Being disabled takes focus, enough focus to get through the most ordinary tasks, focus to handle a job, focus to handle family, focus to forget the tediousness and to remember the spontaneity that allows us laugh deeply. What I discovered I also needed, among the tools of the trade such as crutches, canes, and wheelchairs, was the ability to be open and to be able to talk about my situation honestly, without pathos, without any detrimental emotion.

I became aware that it was my added responsibility to help the able-bodied folks understand what was happening to me, particularly at work, where good communications among coworkers is half of the job. Because my coworkers and I struggled through watching together the changes that occurred in me over a three-year period, we had, fortunately, some time to talk, digest, and assimilate the nature of disability further. After all, able-bodied people have similar needs — needs to understand, needs to help, needs to grow. Because of this commonality, the two-way efforts of communicating together worked. We desired such communication. And we cared.

I did not understand a lot of this in the beginning of my disability. I realize, now, part of communicating well with others involves listening to oneself first, and listening to others really well, then, letting go of all. I also needed to exercise that inner sixth sense, to know what others would tolerate. There were times when I reached out and said, "Look, I know you're scared about what is happening to me, but if you want to talk about it, fine. I promise I will not burst into tears. Also, it's equally okay not to talk." We then usually rapped about things like the weather and the stock market—you know, the life-goes-on stuff.

But, in almost any casual conversation, our vulnerabilities would unexpectedly surface. Unfortunately, like death, our fears and vulnerabilities are taboo subjects in this society. So at the beginning, I needed to reach deep within and share my sense of inner strength. I needed to diminish the scariness so we could face the realities and carry on with work.

Strength, always and in all ways, an admirable quality in people, is not really a matter of discussion, but rather, a felt quality. Likewise, strength is not purchasable. It is developed slowly, cultivated through a myriad of methods: meditation, faith, working with professional help, you name it—and developed experientially. We cannot rush strength. It has its own terms. In giving coworkers confidence that I still had the physical stamina to do the job, I treated work like a marathon. I prepared for it. I rested a lot at home and kept extra-curricular activities to a tolerable minimum. Instead of going out for lunch, I bagged it, relaxed, and meditated during the one-hour lunch break. Much as I wanted to socialize and relax with others, I had other priorities.

I could no longer carry a cup of coffee without spilling half of the contents. So the engineer across the hall brought hot, fresh cups to me. Equally, the other coworkers did not mind pitching in, particularly if they saw me trying to do my share. And I discovered it made them feel good. I did not take advantage of this help. The bottom line was that the job was always my responsibility, always. I never lost sight of that.

Today, I am still very aware and honest about my ability to finish any task. Now, I no longer set superhuman deadlines, but work steadily, utilizing tools such as the computer and organized work habits more than ever. In other words, I still work smarter while being slower. As marketing coordinator for the architectural-engineering firm, I could not, and did not, miss deadlines. My coworkers sensed this dependability and counted on it. The story of the tortoise and hare held, and holds, so true, always and in all ways.

On the job, if I had a shaky day, I exercised humor. It is not a matter of covering up, but a matter of being human: we *all* have shaky days. Laughter, in this case, was an amazing healer and equalizer, very revealing, and graceful. Because I worked on keeping self-consciousness about my disability to a minimum, I joked a lot. Coworkers picked up on this and continued the good-natured joking. In this case, there was no distinction between the disabled and nondisabled.

My boss, meanwhile, got the message. He knew that I'd figure out how to make the deadline, and he exercised wisdom by leaving it to me. I exercised equal wisdom by doing what needed to be done and asking for help if I could not make the deadline. Being very organized was a help in saving energy. Since an unbelievable amount of time was spent walking the halls, I bunched the errands by direction and did them only once or twice a day. Urgent tasks were dealt with via phone.

One of the best bits of advice I got from a senior officer of the firm upon her initially hearing of my situation was, "Karen, learn to use the computer. Become an expert. You can exercise amazing power and skill with this capability." Since I had, and still have, a tremendous amount of respect for this individual, I am always in the process of adding to this skill. As it turns out, there are more and more educational programs specifically for individuals with disabilities to learn computer capabilities—another great equalizer in our lives.

Basic to all of these tactics is the ability to work smart. And working smart happens in the head, not in the body. This axiom affects all working individuals, disabled or not. The late Ken Keyes, disability activist and author of many books such as the *Handbook to Higher Consciousness* and *Your Life Is a Gift,* said shortly before his death, "You create the world with your mind, not your body."

Working smart means, once again, practicing meditation or some form of quieting down. It means clearing the noise and cobwebs from our heads so that we can have the clarity to see what really needs to be done, to be a better player, and to help the team accomplish its tasks. It means sizing up the priorities and realistically fitting them within your capabilities. We were hired, after all, to do just that.

In retrospect, this all sounds easy. It's not. I'm talking about a few years of adjusting, learning, growing, and adjusting some more. I'm referring to the mountain climber's agonizing shortness of breath, to all the women who have had to be 110 percent better to merely realize 80 percent recognition, to the teenager fighting off the temptations of drugs. It's hard, continuously rising above the struggles and continuously reaching out. The successes are small and, most of time, seemingly insignificant. But every time we dare to care, every time we dare to reach out, every time we dare to flex our muscles, we grow.

An interesting thing happened to my boss and me during one of our periodical job reviews. It is an excellent lesson whether you are an employer or employee, with or without a disability. When it comes to a job interview, or on-the-job reviews, our disability, unfortunately, feels more pronounced than ever. We are nervous. It seems that our crutches, canes, wheelchairs, or whatever are more important than the job itself. The anxiety level rises a notch.

During this particular job review, it turned out that my boss was rather nervous. Out of fear of saying the legally wrong thing about my disabling condition, he didn't know how to start the conversation. At the beginning of the review, my disability felt like a third person. It was a situation I had never faced before. The newness of this unexpected challenge made me equally nervous.

Under the Americans with Disabilities Act, any disability is a legal non-issue. However, the reality is that between humans, it is also a matter of familiarity and comfort. How do we deal with that? Here is this person sitting opposite you, a bit tongue-tied, perhaps somewhat paternalistic, or at worst, socially ineffective, and certainly very anxious. The review or interview can go badly, and poof, so can a potential, or existing, job, mostly because of poor communications. What do we do? Legally, we equally don't have to say anything about our conditions.

Realizing that my boss needed to relax, I started talking about myself, my disability, how I was managing day-by-day. Granted, I did not have to say a word about this. But, by opening the door and acknowledging the changes I had encountered the past year, that which both of us had witnessed, I took the initiative to discuss what I was doing to cope. After all, I was responsible for pulling my share to meet the deadlines we all faced as a team.

From this point on, the review continued smoothly. We got down to business, talking about business, talking about how I could help, how he could help, how we could all continue to work together as a team. I spoke of my strengths and weaknesses, and of what I felt I needed to do to carry on. Because we both let our hair down, while remaining professional in approach, the discussions were honest and open. In short, I think my boss walked away from the review with more understanding and familiarity about myself than I ever dreamed. It was a marvelous session.

I realized he knew very little about my condition and was afraid to ask for fear of legal repercussion. So I took the initiative and explained my circumstances matter-of-factly and without pathos. As David Johnson, Presbyterian minister and assistant professor of theology, so well stated in his article, "Who Was That Masked Man?," "When we give people information that they don't have, we lessen their anxiety. And when their anxiety level goes down, so does ours." That is exactly what happened.

For the most part, after any given period, we usually feel normal about our disability. Fine. And, of course, others should feel that way also. That would be fine too. But, the reality is that, in most cases, they have not had the time nor experience to become familiar with our conditions. This unfamiliarity, as well as a myriad of other reasons, unfortunately leads to fear and anxiety. And this creates all the attitudinal barriers that we, persons with disabilities, constantly face. Unfortunately, it is up to us to teach our able-bodied counterparts, to break the barriers, to help them understand our disabilities, to bridge the gap. After all, we are the experts, even though we were hired for some other reason.

SEX

Romance, love, sexual fulfillment, and relationships are universally celebrated, but society still thinks that people with disabilities simply are not capable of or even interested in sex. Up until recently, the taboo around sexuality and disability has been shrouded in silence.

Since I firmly believe all beings are naturally sexual, disabled or not, I am a stout supporter of exploring your sexuality. I also believe there should be no rules—a prime principle that can be deliberated and celebrated by all. Because a shared, solid two-way communication will only serve to deepen your intimacy, it creates a win-win situation all around.

One publication that covers, and covers well, current issues involving dating, communication, intimacy, sexuality, and much more, is *New Mobility*[1] magazine. The message is of a positive and healthy ilk—a read I highly recommend. Another wonderful publication that devotes itself solely to the issue of sexuality and disability is *It's Okay!*,[2] a quarterly magazine published by Sureen Publications and Productions.

I contacted Linda Crabtree, founder of *It's Okay!*, who also is currently involved in another superb organization she founded, the Charcot-Marie-Tooth International,[3] which addresses a form of muscular dystrophy. Regarding *It's Okay!*, she says,

> Since I started *It's Okay!* in 1992, I've seen all
> kinds of inroads made . . . that are taking place,
> *ever so slowly,* as sex and disability is wrestled
> away from the medical profession where it is
> treated as a medical problem (it's no more a
> medical problem for us than it is for able-bodied
> folks) and given back to us who rightly own it so
> we may solve our own problems in our own way
> without interference from those who couldn't
> possibly know how we feel until they've laid in
> our beds.

I also borrow freely the suggestions for topics of discussion from the Swedish booklet, *Sexuality and Disability: A Matter that Concerns All of Us*[4] by Inger Nordqvist printed in 1986 and still very current today. The Swedes are like that: wonderfully open when it comes to issues like sexuality. Needless to say, the topics, found in Appendix C, are applicable to all of us, disabled or not.

To be loved and to love is a universal desire. So, in giving careful thought to our own attitudes and values and in discussing such openly with others can only be beneficial for everyone involved. Doing so will help to dispel myths and misconceptions about sexuality and disability that are so prevalent.

The aforementioned booklet recommends small (no larger than ten persons) study circles concerning issues covering sexuality and disability. Anyone can participate, from the person with a disability to an indirectly involved professional. But as the author of this booklet reminds us,

> It is important that you prepare yourselves, are
> in agreement with what you wish to discuss and
> what you would like to get out of these sessions.

She goes on to advise,

> Try to agree on a common language so that you
> don't talk past each other! There is a tendency to

> talk in very general terms about sex and use
> technical terms instead of [talking] about
> concrete problems. Through techniques such as
> role-playing, you may find it easier to put
> yourself into different situations and understand
> your own and other people's feelings.

And further,

> Discuss some situations where you feel insecure
> and try to deal with them. Continue thinking
> about these matters and talk to other people
> outside your group.

Then, the author recommends discussing the following points, and she asks that you choose which ones hold the highest priority for you.

- Parents' attitude toward the sex life of disabled adolescents.

- How it is to be a parent with a disability.

- Opportunities to meet and daring to look for a partner.

- The fear of losing a partner after becoming disabled.

- Fertility. Contraception. Pregnancy. Childbirth.

- Increased activity on the part of the nondisabled, or the least disabled, partner in the sexual interplay.

- Other sexual activities than intercourse.

- Safe sex.

- AIDS and other sexually transmitted diseases.

- Other sexual orientations such as homosexuality.

Time and time again, the feedback from discussion participants included comments like,

> We wanted factual information around sexual matters. We wanted more frankness. We wanted to make it easier to talk about sexuality and intimate relations. Many of us wanted to know more about the sexual dysfunctions associated with different disabilities and diseases. We wanted to find out what we could do in more concrete terms to make it easier for us to have a good sex life.

And they continued:

> It took quite a long time (about five sessions) before we realized that we had to take time out to discuss our own attitudes. Until we did, we weren't ready to assimilate information about sexual dysfunction . . . [and] the original plan was to disband after ten sessions. But we felt the group had become a support and we had gained a security that we needed. We decided to continue once a month or so and to discuss matters that we felt urgent. We learned that it is important to proceed cautiously and let an atmosphere of mutual trust develop naturally.

Ms. Nordqvist highly recommends going through various kinds of study materials, books, pamphlets, videos and the like. This is where *It's Okay!* becomes useful, as this periodical is constantly reviewing the latest material available concerning sexuality and disability. Ms. Nordqvist suggests offering both positive and negative criticism of the material studied. In doing so, you will discover a great deal about your own attitudes. But the author, in addressing the group leaders, says, "Bear in mind in this context that:

- You can never force your opinion on someone else, either in sexual or other matters.

- You must present information based on facts and emphasize similarities between people with and without disabilities (both groups have heard all too often about the differences).

- Try to create an open and positive atmosphere so that you can start working on whatever negative attitudes exist.

- You must not raise false hopes.

- Show tolerance and understanding for the fact we are all different."

Ms. Nordqvist also stipulates,

> Awareness of one's own values and attitudes toward different forms of sexuality are essential when working to expand the opportunities for [others] to lead a functional sexual life. A few points:
>
> - Think of sexuality as something very broad and not just as sexual intercourse, coitus.
>
> - Give a person who has been injured as an adult back his/her self-confidence and help [this person] discover his/her own sexual identity.
>
> - Be positive and talk about possibilities instead of obstacles.
>
> - Take into consideration the individual's personal values and respect them.
>
> - And do not forget the partner and his/her values concerning sexuality.

Though these suggestions are addressed primarily to group facilitators, they are really points participants should consider. After all, we are helping one another to learn/regain our sexuality.

Ms. Nordqvist claims,

> No professional group is better suited than another to provide information on sexuality and intimate relations. The important thing is to be truly interested, to get your facts straight, and have a desire to do something positive for the good of others.

CHAPTER

20

SUICIDE

For many, it seems that assisted suicide is the answer to having some authority and control over our lives, especially if we have some kind of chronic disease or disability. That is what I thought—for a while, anyway. Then I realized I was buying into the beliefs of others: the better-dead-than-disabled stuff. Whoa, just a minute.

I'm fine as is, thank you. My legs may no longer work, my arms may be weak, I have my off days, and I can no longer drive or feed myself, sooo . . . ? I still laugh, love, cry, contribute, and enjoy a good dessert. I am "not dead yet," the battle cry of the disability community in the wake of the assisted suicide debate.

One question I have is this: who decides who is to die a premature death? In other words, who plays God?

When enduring inexplicable physical pain for over three years, I wanted to put an end to it—and to my life—since I was not getting any relief from the traditional medical world. It was a good thing I decided to endure a bit longer. I finally found help through an alternative healing method. Granted, the search for help took over two years while I was also seeking relief by the traditional route. Fortunately, the search ended when I was at my wits end, being both quite desperate and exhausted. In this case, the timing was all. Hindsight now tells me I would have played a lousy Goddess then. Being in such a state of mind could have resulted in any unclear move, the pain coloring all. Based on this experience, if I were to play Goddess now, there are a couple of things I would say .

First, we need to stop judging others. I mean, who is to put a value on life, on *anyone's* life, for that matter? Second, let's put a greater emphasis on palliative care—that is, relieving the pain which can be either physical or emotional—not on deciding when to end life. In other words, let's follow former President George Bush's advice and become a kinder and gentler society by finding better ways to alleviate pain—pain that can be either physical or emotional.

A case in point: Wouldn't it be different if a doctor were to say, "Look, I identify with the pain you are in, and though I'm unable to deal with the source of that, I plan to partner with you in creating relief. And I intend to be at your side throughout." Wouldn't that be a lot different?

Finding better means of easing pain is something western medicine is not doing well at all. Instead, the emphasis is on how to prolong life, not on how to make it easier to live, even if we're dying. And, of course, with today's current medical trend toward "managed care," any palliative treatment is becoming even less important.

Understandably, our fear of death is not so much of the dying in itself as much as it is of dying in a strange hospital room connected to a bunch of tubes and wires primarily meant to keep us, at all cost, painfully alive. Simply, I wonder what our transition would be like if doctors, and other individuals, would take an effort to make us as comfortable as humanly possible so we could die a natural, and dignified, death. I feel, in part, that if this were emphasized, the support for assisted suicide would flounder.

A very real anxiety the disability community has is the voiceless, silent decision on who dies—a very real fear. Remember, people with disabilities (PWDs) were some of Hitler's earliest victims. And the doctors doing this thought they were being "patriotic." Patriotic? Maybe that is what they thought, but hindsight clearly stipulates that they were murderers. What is so scary about this is the amount of hatred and naiveté floating around our country today. These feelings are not really much different than those that were drifting around in Germany's pre-Hitler days before World War II. And sadly, much as I love the Netherlands—having traveled to Holland a few times and having become quite fond of some individuals living there—I am very disturbed by what is happening in that country.

Holland is the first, and to date the only, nation in the world to legalize assisted suicide. Following the old saying, "If you want to know what's down the road, then ask those coming back," we certainly can learn from the Dutch, their having been down the road. According to a July 21, 1996, *New York Times Magazine* article, "The Next Pro-Lifers," author Paul Wilkes clearly lays out the problems of legalizing assisted suicide in reference to Holland's experience.

Wilkes writes about psychiatrist Herbert Hendin, among other individuals. Hendin first traveled to the Netherlands in 1993 specifically to study the assisted suicide phenomenon there. Subsequently, Hendin wrote a book on the subject, *Seduced by Death* (1996, W.W. Norton). Hendin says in this book, "Virtually every guideline established by the Dutch to regulate euthanasia has been modified or violated with impunity." That's scary. To wit, an article in *Mouth* magazine's November-December 1996 issue reports that in 1990 over an estimated 11,000 disabled people were euthanized *without their consent*. How did this happen? The doctors made a judgment and determined the worthiness, or lack thereof to be more precise, of their patients' lives. And because assisted suicide—read that as terminating life—is sanctioned in Holland, theoretically no one was doing anything legally wrong.

Scary. In this gray area, this loophole, someone is making a judgment. Someone is playing God/Goddess/Buddha/whatever. I didn't know laws created and condoned that. In fact, I would never allow an elected politician to sanctify an individual to determine if my life is worth living or not.

It is precisely at this juncture that PWDs have ample grounds to worry. Our lives are being judged constantly by others. And their perceptions, nine times out of ten, are so very different than ours. Assorted polls demonstrate just how large the perception gap is. On a scale of one to ten, the highest number being the best, doctors would place a value on the quality of a PWD's life. The numbers would run especially low if that person used a respirator, day, night, or anytime. Conversely, PWDs rated themselves as placing much more value on their lives, of experiencing more life satisfaction than the doctors, or anyone for that matter, would perceive. Even I have personally experienced this tremendous gap of perception. Needless to say, I remain quite flabbergasted. And scared.

I wouldn't trust a court-sanctioned doctor to place a value on my life. Would you? So I worry. If assisted suicide were legalized, would my life be snuffed out by someone who perceives my life as not worth living simply because it is "different" from what is considered the norm? Think about this. It is highly possible. You may say, "Oh, safeguards will take care of that." I ask, "After six plus years, why has Holland not yet accomplished this?" I worry. This silent decision-making is murder if you ask me.

Mary Frances Platt, a writer and disability activist, astutely observes, "Like racism, ableism can be subtle or overt, and in the case of growing support of assisted suicide in the United States, it is life threatening." So I worry. And if I quietly disappear, I think you should be worried too. Let the concern not be hindsight. Let it not be silent.

PART THREE

On Becoming Savvy
and Then Some

21

MENTORS, MENTORSHIP, AND OTHER ADMIRALS

When I first started using the wheelchair, my angels must have been working, pulling strings of every sort. Within the first year of wheelchair use, I met Ed Roberts, father of the independent living movement, and two other activists in the disability community who have had an extremely powerful and lasting effect on me. These other two disability activists both took me under their wings—a changing of angel guardians, so to speak. They provided an immediate sense of disability pride and cool. They equally gave an immediate understanding of how to be gently political. Ironically, in losing the stride I had walking about on my own two legs, I never lost stride rolling about in my chair with these folks. They both were adamant about resolving the injustices the disability community carried, yet, when being with them, they could have been wearing T-shirts saying, "I'm disabled, sooo . . . ?"

In 1989, when I first met Dr. Adolf Ratzka, a renowned disability activist living in Stockholm, Sweden, I was just beginning to use a wheelchair. During my six-week stay in Stockholm, I visited Adolf and his wife as much as I could. Over time, my association with Adolf still remains special. I also discovered the highest meaning of the axiom, "There is no such thing as a coincidence. It is God being anonymous."

Adolf was born in Bavaria, Germany. His family came from Czechoslovakia. He finished his studies in California and got a Ph.D. in Economics from the University of California at Los Angeles. He then relocated to Sweden, married, and eventually adopted a baby girl. Adolf travels worldwide, primarily covering disability issues, continues to write, gives speeches, and remains very involved in the disability community, locally, regionally, and internationally. On our last visit, I interviewed Adolf. And learned a lot. Here is a small part of our two-hour talk. What he has to say here are words of wisdom, whether you use a wheelchair or are an able-bodied person going through a divorce.

Karen Stone: Tell me, how and when did you first became disabled?

Adolf Ratzka: I became disabled when I was seventeen years old and in high school. Due to polio, I spent the next five years in a hospital institution until I was twenty-three. That was a very important time in my life, and I am still upset about the missed years, which actually put me back. In the hospital, you are really exposed to the brutal totalitarian system. Even the nicest people have to follow the rules which end up limiting your life, and it can break you personally. In an institution where there is nothing to say, then there is no way you can control your life or you can keep your spirit alive. It is very dehumanizing and degrading.

KS: When you say, "It can break you," how did you sustain yourself?

AR: I was extremely lucky. I was encouraged to continue school. I had high hopes of going to the U.S. for my education. I planned almost every minute for the "Big Exam." I knew that if I didn't get the highest grades on the test, I wouldn't get the scholarship.

KS: Is that what kept you alive?

AR: My hope was to escape and make up for all of this in California. This was my dream. I knew about the sun and beaches. I got a full scholarship from the state of Bavaria and that paid my way all through school until I received my Ph.D.

KS: Let's address the activism you now do on an international level. Can you talk more about that?

AR: Well, in my experiences here and abroad, I couldn't help drawing the conclusion that the disabled are second-class citizens wherever they lived. It seemed to me in the beginning that I could avoid the second-class citizenship by excelling in my field. But, I also lived for five years in an institution and there was this undercurrent fear of people putting me back. You think, "Once a prisoner, always a prisoner."

KS: What do you have to say about the personal and the political?

AR: My professional life is now centered around disability. If someone gave me a pill and said, "Now you can walk again," I'd be in bad shape because I would have to re-identify myself. This would take years. My asset is being able to put the personal and political together because of my circumstances.

KS: Any final words?

AR: You look around and see other people living halfway. They are missing something. They have nothing to work for, to live for. They do not have a self-giving, self-evident, natural, immediate cause. But in our case, it is quite obvious. I do not have to search for a meaning in life. Fighting for myself is also fighting for the world.

Five years after meeting Adolf, I was hoping for an un-eventful end to 1993. Wrong. I learned that disability activist and former Albuquerque resident, Dr. Kirk MacGugan, had died. She was my other guardian angel. So I found myself writing a eulogy, something very difficult for me to do.

I am shocked by your death, Kirk.

Getting polio at the age of twelve before the arrival of the Salk vaccine, you grew up in Hatch, New Mexico. And ended up in Albuquerque with husband, Tommy, in 1986, where you worked toward a second doctorate at University of New Mexico, this time in history. Now it's all history . . .

A few years ago, when I saw your newly purchased bright red power wheelchair, I thought how chic, how Sally Raphaelish. But Sally Raphael notwithstanding, you would have gotten a red-colored power chair anyway . . .

I remember you and Tommy going through throes of wanting and coming close to adopting a child. I don't think you ever stopped wanting to have a child, so full of love you were . . .

I remember giving a talk to one of the classes you were teaching while obtaining your doctorate. It was then I had the wonderful privilege of watching you interface with your students. So full of respect and love they were for you . . .

You taught without being didactic that the political is personal, no matter how you cut it. There could be no way of experiencing disability and being apolitical. Your activism was professional, polished, pointed, and yet, gentle. You genuinely affected the many friends, co-workers, political cohorts, students, and more, you came in contact with.

I remember the long, hot afternoons and summer eve-nings at your Corrales abode or at the Pinto Restau-rant, sharing jokes and war stories. One, in particular, was when you were first driving with the then available crude hand controls and the brake mechanism failed.

You tried lifting your uncooperative leg onto the foot brake, but that proved to be rather impossible while driving a brakeless automobile. Being close to home and on a straight run, you managed to make it directly up the driveway—and finally crashed into a bunch of garbage cans to come to a stop. We had a hearty laugh over the value of garbage cans. But, in reality, that was your style of doing things—head-on. In true manner, you were just like what your license plate said: Admiral.

When I first entered the disability world, you took me under your wing. You gave and demonstrated to me that there is definitely life after a wheelchair . . .

I am not alone with these memories. You affected an untold number of people, both here in New Mexico and in San Francisco where you have been the last couple of years.

In your last days, dear friend Beatriz Mitchell says of you, "When Kirk was hospitalized in San Francisco, her many friends started to visit . . . Tommy said that her room and the hospital halls were crowded with people, with and without wheelchairs, waiting in line to see Kirk. Finally the hospital staff asked that Tommy send them home. They were disrupting the running of the hospital!"

Kirk, you lit all our fires and kept them going, while being both the match and the fuel. You gave so much. Beatriz says, "She saw the greatness in all of us and expected us to reach our calling. There is an epitaph on Coleridge's tombstone that reads, 'He touched nothing that he did not adorn.'"

I went out into the garden and grieved.

Then, though not a direct guardian angel of mine, but more of an acquaintance, Ed Roberts of Oakland, California, died of an apparent heart attack on March 14, 1995. Ed was the very man who said at one of Kirk's many memorial services, "If you hadn't been married to Tommy, I would have married you!" He was fifty-six. Once again, I found myself in the garden grieving. And wrote:

> The feeling among the disability community is one of shock and great sadness. The loss that comes with Ed Roberts' death is, and will be, for years, acutely felt. Ed was not simply a slumbering giant of the invisible, but an initial part of the powerful, disability rights movement that has rocked nations worldwide. He was, to many, disabled or not, far more. Ed Roberts was a Martin Luther King of the disability rights movement.

> At the ripe age of fourteen, Ed nearly died of polio. As a result, the attending doctor said if Ed were to survive, he would be a vegetable the rest of his life. Upon hearing those words, Ed decided he would be his favorite vegetable—an artichoke. So, leaf by leaf, Ed unfolded. Sleeping in an iron lung at night, and getting around during the day in his power wheelchair provided with a respirator, Ed moved through the educational ranks by phone until he was ready to enter the University of California (UC), Berkeley, in the early 1960s.

> As writer Joseph P. Shapiro says in his book on the disability rights movement in the United States, *No Pity* (1993, Random House), "Just as surely as [James] Meredith ushered in an era of access to higher education for blacks and a new chapter in civil rights movement, Roberts was quietly opening a civil rights movement that would remake the world for disabled people. The disability rights movement was born the day Roberts arrived on the Berkeley campus."

> It was there at the Berkeley campus that the system tried to stop Roberts. UC said he was too disabled for the university to accommodate him. California's Department of Vocational Rehabilitation (DVR) would not fund his education. They considered Ed too disabled to be educated or employed. Like all fearless leaders, Ed would not accept a rejection. Ed declared he could, and would, with appropriate assistance, attend the university. Not able to accommodate his eight-

hundred-pound iron lung in any campus dormitory, Ed spent his evenings within his iron lung at the university's Cowell Hospital, very alone.

Hiring individuals to attend to his personal needs, and joined by other members of the disability community, Ed became one of the "Rolling Quads" on campus and a well-known activist. Ed was on campus studying political science during the Free Speech Movement and the anti-Vietnam-War protests. During these formative years, Ed not only received his bachelor's and master's in political science, but began working on his doctor's degree as well.

By the fall of 1970, with a grant from the Department of Health, Education, and Welfare, Roberts and the Rolling Quads started the Physically Disabled Students' Program (PDSP) on campus. The rest is history. Close to over a decade after being called "unfeasibly employable" by California's DVR, Ed was hired by the then Governor, Jerry Brown, to be the Department of Vocational Rehabilitation director.

Taking the seemingly contradictory activities of independent living and rehabilitation services, Ed instead created a marriage between the two. He realigned DVR's funding focus, which had been on rehabilitation, to one that would lend itself more to independent lifestyles. As with the PDSP, criteria such as self-sufficiency, independence, and mainstreaming became the benchmark of DVR's work. He held the DVR position until 1982.

All along, Ed never considered his disability a problem. He always considered disability a social dilemma. Recognized for his work in the disability arena, Ed was honored by the MacArthur Foundation in 1984. With their monetary gift, Ed co-founded the World Institute on Disability. And the ripples of his work in the disability rights movement spread worldwide.

So now, we members of the visibly growing disability community are it. There is no longer an Ed Roberts to pull and push us along, to inspire us—to use the very words that would make him frown. We are it. We need to show the world, the MacArthur Foundation, DVR, our sons and daughters, and our next-door neighbor that disability is really in the minds of others. There lies our true challenge.

Ed, thank you so much. These words are a far cry from what you have meant and done for us. I'll never forget your sense of humor and clarity of purpose in life. This everlasting gift I will carry with me always and in all ways. They say, "If you are disabled, you don't go heaven when you die. Instead, you go to Berkeley." Ed, you are largely responsible for making Berkeley a heaven of sorts. May you rest there in peace, knowing that we will carry your banner of independence to the rest of the world.

There is a Chinese proverb, "To know the road ahead, ask those coming back." For many of us, we need to ask. We need mentors. Surprisingly, for some, we are already offering a role model to others without even knowing. Too, the list of those that are blazing the mentorship trails need not be set forth here. We often hear about such individuals.

But what is crucial to all this is understanding that all of us carry some responsibility in letting those who follow our tracks know that life does continue beyond having a disability. This is a demonstration of mentorship, so to speak. And we carry the responsibility to let others know that we equally share the burden of making our world better; to let others know that they are not alone.

Of course, there is always work involved in improving things, and we round our shoulders in carrying the load. Susan Nussbaum, an actor, playwright and a disability rights activist describes the importance of such work:

> The peace movement, sexism, rights for the
> disabled—none of these are isolated issues.
> They're not glitches, they're part of a pattern.
> Some of the most progressive political work
> that's happening in this country is in the area of
> disability rights. It cuts across ideology, age and

> race differences and inspires such raw, all-out
> courage from people who figure they've got
> nothing left to lose.

In considering this, you probably are thinking of all the work that still needs to be done. And round your shoulders even more. Too, you probably never thought of yourself as a mentor. Yet, in ways, we all are. We look to one another for the much-needed esprit de corps. We look to each other for humanity, the chance to simply be ourselves, the chance to laugh, cry, and drink a cup of tea, the chance to be human and not to be a "super crip." The old, oft-said axiom, "There is power in numbers," undoubtedly offers us comfort here. And then some.

As many of you know, being a mentor involves being comfortable with who you are. People are drawn to comfort. A large part of being comfortable is acceptance — acceptance of ourselves as we are and acceptance of others as they are. Another quality found in mentors is that of egolessness. Such individuals are beyond themselves, beyond the "I," the "me," the "mine"-ness of things. A wheelchair may be part of the picture, but so what. Life is greater than chairs, and mentors focus on this very livingness, on the greater picture, and not on any of the limitations.

Too, we are drawn to those who take themselves lightly. Remember the saying, "Angels can fly because they take themselves lightly." Of course, being disabled is no easy burden. But it seems that the individuals who become role models have broken through this personal barrier. The ability to laugh at ourselves, our predicaments, helps. I just returned from a week-long seminar for persons with disabilities. A very enjoyable moment turned out to be a hilarious round-table, story-telling session of our most embarrassing falls.

It helps to make others laugh as well. So wearing a Groucho Marx bushy-mustache, enlarged-nose pair of glasses to meetings is entirely appropriate. But the humor doesn't end with our taking the glasses off. Like angels, we must continue to fly — while wearing our glasses and then some.

You are probably thinking, "Yeah, sure, with the burden of my disability, the constant burden of oppression, the endless work that needs doing, and more, *how* am I to fly with *that* load? !" Well, there is always the need for a certain amount of optimism. Novelist and essayist Wallace Stegner, upon discussing examples of optimism, says,

> We shouldn't allow ourselves to be rendered
> inert, like the octopus that couldn't decide
> which leg to use while in a bowl of milk, so he
> sat in the middle of his legs and drowned.

Stegner prefers the frog who found himself trapped in this bowl of milk. Against all reason, the frog kept swimming, until the milk had turned to butter and allowed him to climb out.

PARKING, WARS,
AND OTHER BATTLES

Life is a challenge? So is the ordinary daily round. Think about it. A trip to the nearby mall can be full of challenges. First, the person with a disability drives around and around the parking lot, looking for a place to park. All the handicap parking spaces are filled, more than half by people illegally doing so. You know who you guilty ones are.

Finally, this person sees a space. But no! Someone has parked in the adjoining striped area where no one is suppose to park. Why the stripes? So a person has space on the side for the van's wheelchair lift or ramp to operate. So she ends up parking alongside the main entry of the parking lot where she has ample room to open and lower her lift, all at the risk of being hit by an approaching car. It happened once — and she got the ticket for being in an improper area, despite her broken wheelchair and collarbone. On top of all, to get to the mall, she still has to go behind the many parked cars between her and the main entrance of the mall. This requires being on super alert. Drivers, when backing out, usually cannot see someone so low in a wheelchair.

209

At last inside, she hunts for an accessible rest room. Accessible it is marked, and truly accessible it is not. Though wide enough, the door is too heavy to open. Someone has to do it for her. She washes her hands with water only, the soap being too far back to sufficiently reach. And then, she dries her hands on her Levi's, the towel rack too high, alas, to reach.

At the bookstore, she cannot get back to the gardening book section, because the day's *Wall Street Journal, U.S.A. Today,* and local papers are heaped on the floor until the clerk can stack them away on shelves. So without being able to look at her selection, she asks the clerk to bring her the books. Unknown to both of them, he misses a few. And sitting in the front area where the traffic is busy, the customer has no sense of leisure for choosing her selection.

Finally, mission accomplished, she leaves. And repeats the parking lot scenario with the long roll back to her van. Only this time, she is a bit wetter due to an unexpected cloudburst.

Does it sound like I am exaggerating here? I'm not. Though the character in the story may be anyone with a disability, the incidents are true. There is no end to meeting challenges. For persons with any kind of disability, endurance, patience, and humor is a must, even if for a few hours. The standard one-hour trip to the mall becomes a three-hour expedition. It is the norm.

The "handicap parking" (HP) spaces are being used by all sorts of people, including a large number of those having no disability whatsoever. Recently, on the television program, "48 Hours," there was a segment on the issue of people illegally using HP spaces in San Francisco. Because parking is at a premium there, these HP spaces are highly coveted by nonqualified users. In fact, there is even a growing black market among the nondisabled population to buy stolen handicap placards. In some cities, these illegal parkers are called "parking hogs." Most appropriate.

This problem is, and has been, endemic across the entire United States. No place is immune. To wit, many cities now are getting stricter with their police enforcement, fines, and any supporting public patrolling programs as well. It is not that persons with disabilities have chosen such headaches. These spaces have been earmarked primarily for the *safety* of persons with disabilities, not for people to fight over.

The biggest hazard for persons with disabilities when they must park elsewhere is the risk of being hit while rolling, limping, or whatever on their way to a main entrance. Being so low to the ground in our wheelchair means that drivers simply don't see us. Being a slow walker means there is no time to jump aside. Dealing with an environmental illness means being very sensitive to automobile pollution while walking any distance. Such an exposure can result in five days in bed to recover.

Again, this is not an issue of privilege. It is a safety factor. If it were safe, and for some, easy enough to go any distance, persons with disabilities of course would park anywhere just like anyone else. But, there have been too many horror stories about persons with disabilities being forced to park elsewhere with dreadful consequences.

So some cities are, or have been, creating "handicap parking enforcement programs," also known as "citizen patrolling units." Frustrated citizens, disabled or not, have signed up, been trained by the local police department, have canvassed hot spots—like mall parking lots during peak hours—and have issued citations with fines commonly $100, some now as high as $250. So these volunteers are busy. To wit, a volunteer patrolling citizen of the Broward County Sheriff's Department, near Ft. Lauderdale, Florida, says, ". . . at one Pompano Beach shopping center, sixty-three people illegally parked in spaces reserved for 'the handicapped' in just five hours." Numbers like this are very common.

The volunteers see their task as a labor of love. Speaking of these volunteers, the Broward County Sheriff's Department says, "They have experienced, first hand, the frustration of seeing an able-bodied motorist drive into a parking space clearly marked 'handicapped only.'" The Sheriff's Department established Broward County's citizen patrolling unit years ago, in 1986.

Take, for another example, the city of Denver. About their handicapped parking enforcement program, the Denver Police Department says, "This program is not designed to punish offenders but to foster awareness . . ."

According to numerous reports, cities that already have established these programs, mostly staffed by well-trained volunteers, report virtually no disturbing incidents so far. This is a statement that people appreciate being educated or reminded. Repeat offenders, like students who "borrow" their grandmother's placard for university campus parking, deserve any fine imposed by any city. They are not only creating safety barriers, but are blocking an individual's access to education. This simply is intolerable.

There are also the other illegal parkers who say "Hey, I am only going to be here a minute." But in being forced to park elsewhere, all it takes is one second for yours truly to be clobbered by a car. Again, we are talking about safety, not privilege.

Meanwhile, some other battles . . .

Recently, a very well known disk jockey on a local radio station told the following joke: "What's the difference between Christopher Reeves and O.J. Simpson? O.J. will walk." Like myself, everyone I repeated this to reacted with utter distaste. That this radio station would allow such a joke to be aired is extremely unhealthy. It breeds prejudice. And prejudice is the precursor to hate.

Such distasteful jokes fly in the very face of our understanding the "other." We need to learn to live alongside persons with a disability, people of color, women, with anyone. How? To realize that the "other" is not "they," but us, all of us, is a big step in the right direction. Ironically, the very person who told this joke on the radio can become disabled anytime. He can be innocently clobbered by a drunken driver on his way home from work. As has been often said, disability is a club anyone can join, anytime, anywhere, Superman or not. We all have our differences, difficulties, or challenges.

These very qualities create our common bond, our common heritage, the glue of humankind. We all laugh, cry, and pay taxes. So what if a wheelchair or a pair of glasses becomes an appendage in our lives. Do you treat someone unkindly because they need to use glasses? The Simpson/Reeves joke definitely does not point the way to raise our children.

Prejudice leads to hate and hate breeds conflicts. Conflicts often result in war. Then everyone loses. What a lousy deal. There are innocent children, women, and men dying overseas due to war. Also, there are those who are surviving, surviving the terror, surviving the loss of loved ones, surviving with injuries.

Here in America, in time of war, some individuals return intact. Some come back in body bags. And some will return with a disability. This comes with war. It is one of those lousy marriages. This crummy union hits our home front very hard, any home front hard. Your once able-bodied son or daughter may be that very person who returns with a permanent injury. Or it may be your niece, nephew, neighbor. It may be your friend. Or husband. Or wife. It can be anyone. You never thought it would happen, and poof—what can I say? You are probably asking the same.

Yet, the veterans returning with disabling injury endure far more pain than necessary. Need we welcome those back from some war-torn territory with blatant biases about people with disabilities? Need the people returning from any war with a permanent injury endure this added, and unnecessary, pain? No. And believe me, you can help.

Upon returning home, these individuals, like you and me, will have plans to carry on. That is to be expected, injury not withstanding. Some will attend college, some are part of a family, some plan to get married, to raise children, to work— to do just as before. In that regard, nothing has changed. How can you make things more graceful at this awkward time? A few suggestions follow.

Understand that people with disabilities are really no different than anyone else. We still need to wash our dirty socks. We still need to get the grocery shopping done. At movies, we still find ourselves laughing and crying. We vote, plan, and dream like everyone else. Like children, we love to play.

We are students. We pay taxes, we love cappuccinos, and we enjoy an afternoon at the zoo.

Understand that those of us with mobility problems feel very handicapped by the physical barriers out there, not by our wheelchairs, if we are using one. Understand that our chairs are simply mobility devices the way glasses are seeing devices for others. So refuse to honor businesses that refuse to honor wheelchairs and the like. Speak out and let the owner or manager know why you are no longer going there.

In the same vein, make sure that community activities are accessible (see Appendix A). Undoubtedly, this will encourage greater participation of people with disabilities. In the mingling, we all make contact. And in this contact, we will further dispel disparaging myths. Understand that we individuals with disabilities like to mix, to mainstream, to be with anyone at any time, and not necessarily just be among members of the disability community.

One important common courtesy relates to personal privacy. You don't ask people about their incomes or sex lives. Likewise, it is not very kosher for an adult to ask somebody about their disability. On the other hand, I do welcome questions from children. They are open, inquisitive, funny, and very accepting. As previously mentioned, children have a natural, uninhibited curiosity and ask questions that some adults might find embarrassing. Scolding kids for asking such questions may make them think there is something "bad" about having a disability.

There is more. Much more. This is a small start. War and disability, a lousy marriage, is a marriage we cannot ignore. It is here to stay. And it is up to all of us to help any injured individual returning home to readjust, even in small ways—remember the Talmud saying, "If you help one, you help the world."

MONEY AND CHANGE

Over the past few years, I have gone from being able to walk to being unable to fully dress myself. Quite a change. It takes so long to do everything now, but then, what is time? They say, "Time is money." But then, what is money?

A lot, especially to a person with a disability. As I stated in Chapter 2, the lack of money can be a formidable barrier to independent living. I spend all my discretionary income and savings on disability products or personal assistance to simply to make life somewhat more manageable, while maintaining an independent status. But I must confess that such a constant financial outlay is getting a bit tiring. Yet, as my upper torso became affected by my condition, I installed a barrier-free ceiling lift. Without upper body strength to transfer, for example, from the wheelchair to shower seat, I need assistance. So I bought a lift and spent $6,000. This, unfortunately, is in part the price of independence.

But, for me, it is worth every cent. Now my wake-up call is the shower. What an unmitigated luxury. I no longer have to wait until 11 A.M. for the necessary strength to take a shower. What a physical and mental luxury. Nor, with this lift on hand, do I have to schedule my bladder. Too, no longer does anyone else have to hurt their back in helping out. But, the changes continue. I install an $800 low-effort power steering unit in my car, while hoping that accessible public transportation becomes the norm before the car, or myself, wears out.

I'd like to get a power wheelchair, the manual chair turning out to be a bit difficult to push now. I saw one at the Abilities Expo. Price tag? $5,000. And that's on the cheap side. When, oh when, does it end? Savings are nil; for a long time, I refused to go on Medicaid; and my HMO does not provide these things. Any government assistance comes with phenomenal red tape, paperwork, and frustration. The squeeze between being poor, begging, or being rich enough to buy independence is challenging, mildly put.

It is no wonder my disabled brothers and sisters feel so exploited. It is not cheap to become or to be disabled, and to remain independent. In fact, in most of the world, there is not even a choice for many persons with a disability about such matters. This makes me think of the persons with disabilities from South Africa, Brazil, Lithuania, and more that I met at the Independence '92 conference in Vancouver, Canada. Their stories have shattered my heart. I count my blessings over and over again.

Since at least a third of our nation does not have medical insurance, many of us have to fork out a great deal for tools to assist us in living any sort of independent lifestyle. Because of this, our savings usually are depleted.

There are power wheelchairs that average $7,000 to $8,000 each. Beyond the older manual wheelchairs, often referred to as "tanks," the more maneuverable lightweight models cost a minimum of $2,000 each. Along the same line, getting an adapted vehicle usually involves the cost of the van, plus an extra $15,000 to convert it with a raised roof or lowered floor, hand controls, and a lift or ramp to get in. I will not even venture to specify the costs of remodeling a home for accessibility.

However, following this line of thought, remodeling expenses could be partially alleviated by building all new homes with accessible, and not obvious, built-in features such as three-foot, six-inch interior doors instead of the standard thirty-inch width, no floor level changes, or a bigger bathroom on the first level. It costs very little to make these adjustments on the drawing board. But after the fact, in retrofitting a built structure, you pay. Mightily.

For a person living with a chronic illness, the cost of drugs, western medical treatment, or alternative care can add up. For those that have a hearing difficulty, communication devices are not cheap. For a person who needs a prosthesis, count your dollars. On top of it all, in many cases, there is no Ralph Nader on the scene to monitor quality vs. quacks.

There are also maintenance costs for equipment. One little horror story signifies just how expensive this can be. The belt from the motor to the rear axle of my motorized rickshaw cost $30 alone. A neighbor put it in, saving me a minimum $35 for the labor to install. Meanwhile, Pep Boys charges $7.99 for an automobile fan belt. . . . Who pays for the added difference? I do.

I have been talking to a number of doctors about affordable health care, doctors in private practice, doctors from the public sector, and those working within HMOs. No other issue in the United States economy seems less understood than affordable health care. Affordable health is, but should not be, a confusing proposition. And it involves all of us. In this case, there is no "us" versus "them." The problem of good health care for everyone at a reasonable cost is a quagmire that we all agonize over, disabled or not.

Despite blatant inequities, we spent an estimated $700 billion in 1995 on health care. That's twelve percent of our total economy. That's $2,700 per American. We'll spend as much on health care this year as on cars and trucks, plus gasoline and parts. Persons with disabilities spend more.

The Office of Trade and Economic Analysis says that by one of their indicators, our personal savings have gone from 8 percent in 1970 to 4.8 percent in 1992. Meanwhile, our medical costs were 7.4 percent of our gross domestic products

(GDP) in 1970 and 13.2 percent of the GDP in 1991, as reported in late 1992 by the U.S. Health Care Financing Administration.

Countries that have universal health care, such as Germany and Japan, realize an average personal savings two and a half times greater than ours, according to the U.S. Department of Commerce. So it can be concluded that our medical costs have some impact on our savings. What a dismal thought.

Many people living with a disability personally fork out a great deal for tools to assist in living any sort of independent lifestyle. Because of this, as previously mentioned, our savings usually are depleted. Let me repeat what a friend said, when talking about no savings, "There is nothing between you and the big, bad wolves out there." Another dismal thought.

Being proactive about preventative health care measures such as education in good eating, explaining the effects of fetal alcohol syndrome, or exercising on a regular basis is financially beneficial. I tried, along with my doctor, to get my HMO, which advocates *preventative* health care, to provide a workout space for people with special needs. No luck. Instead, the existing gyms only are for people on the mend in physical therapy. A lousy and expensive way to practice preventative health care, if you ask me.

Monitoring third-party payment systems can help to keep the fat profits at bay. Because these bills are often paid for by Medicaid, Medicare, or private insurance, price tags are rarely questioned. There simply is no check and control. The bill gets bigger every month. Who pays? We all do.

According to one doctor, this quagmire is affecting more and more people. He even sees an increase of the able-bodied middle class utilizing the services of our local university hospital, services that are either low-cost or free. But actually, these services are not really free. We support this hospital in part with tax money. Despite the clamor for change, there is no agreement on what change to pursue. According to one doctor from my HMO, he feels we need to spend more health care money on education. He says, "The best way to spend money is to get people to quit smoking, to work on drug and alcohol abuse, to increase awareness of preventative health care practices."

According to another doctor in private practice, the risk of a malpractice suit hovers over his good will, and such risk is the result of continuing problems in our health care system. He says,

> I can try to help by seeing a person free of charge, and that person may misread the prescription and possibly under or overdose on the medication. My return for kindness? A malpractice suit, even though it is not my fault.

CHAPTER

24

THE LAST STOP

In October, 1995, I wrote:

> At least the walls are not green. And the food is better than your typical institutional variety. The floor staff is extraordinarily hard-working, loving, and committed. To make an unbelievable story short, I am regrouping in a nursing home, not unwell enough to be in a hospital, but not well enough to remain at home. Hopefully by the time you are reading this, I'll be back home.

> When my case worker initially brought up the idea of my going to a nursing home, I nearly had a grand mal seizure. A nursing home!? In my books, it is the ultimate no-no. Then, I was told my family in California was worried, mildly put. So I consented. The last thing in the world I want to do is put my family through any unnecessary emotional gymnastics. But, a nursing home? ? ? ! ! !

> Nursing homes are a no-no among members of the disability community. And with reason. Many persons with disabilities are inappropriately placed in nursing homes, simply because there is no other place to go. And persons with disabilities in nursing homes are like

fish out of water. Look at my current situation. At forty-eight, I am the baby of this place. No fun.

Remember the incredibly poignant closing scene in the movie, *Driving Miss Daisy,* that took place in a nursing home dining hall? Well, it is what I saw here every day. To avoid witnessing the painfully sad scene and to avoid dealing with any subsequent tears, I ate either in my room or out in the courtyard. Alone. I also ate alone to avoid publicity. I thought I was safe from the recognition factor, my coming here under a different name. But, I needed more, like a wig and then some, in order to remain completely anonymous. By the second day, word got back to me that the floor staff knew who occupied room 105 and they were nervous.

So I promptly went to the director and said, "Look, you have the staff treat me like everyone else or you treat everyone else like me." This place is reputed to be the best nursing home in Albuquerque, "in the state," so they claim. I cannot judge, having so little experience with nursing homes here.

What I can say is what often is said about any big business. It is time to exercise creative management. It is time to break down the traditional hierarchical—and often patriarchal—system a bit. In fact, when you think about it, creative management has never hurt a business. Any business. Any time. Any place. It goes without saying, managers should work on the floor at least one day a month in order to get a feel for all that goes on.

Working under tremendous loads, the floor staff maintains volumes of equanimity and offers a very personal touch at the same time. It is precisely because of this that this place has such a fine reputation. I wonder how much management acknowledges such. Sure, there are the sour lemons, the rough, invisible handlers—invisible as long as "20/20"s hidden cameras are not here to record all as they did in their nursing home horror show a few weeks back. Unfortunately, lousy workers come with the territory.

At least it does not feel like any of the staff members have criminal records as proven so prevalent in nursing homes on the aforementioned "20/20" show. But you wonder not only about that and about the management, but also about the owners' motives. There is obviously a profit squeeze-play going on in this place.

To wit, this place feels like it operates with a skeletal floor staff on all shifts. So overloaded are they that to respond to a call within twenty minutes is an amazing feat. Occasionally, it was faster, but rarely. Yet, my family paid top dollar for my stay.

No surprise. During the financially stressful year of 1993, the American Health Care Association trade journal, the *Provider*, reported profits for nursing homes to be up twenty-one percent that year. Based on figures reported in the Merrill Dow Long-term Care report, the average nursing home made approximately $6,300 per patient that year. And who pays? Patients and/or their families, taxpayers, and the floor staff who work extremely hard at low wages. Who wins? No comment.

A nursing home—the place people often call "the last stop" and with good reason. Indeed, almost any nursing home is a scary place, a place where you lose all your autonomy and sense of well-being, if not any actual wellness that you may have left. Let's face it: nursing homes simply are not health spas.

It was not until returning to my own environment that I realized how deep my descent into utter dependency became. Deep and steep. And very scary. But, to be fair, I needed the rest, and not having the megabucks to go to a health spa—which, of course, I would prefer—I went to a nursing home simply because there was no other place to go. No other place—that is the scary part, especially for one who is not that old and has a disability.

The foundation of this future blueprint is not pretty, nor very strong. I happened to hear the following from my neighbor. Her mother was at the same nursing home in which I was residing, and the family chose to pull her from that very nursing home the day after my arrival there. Their reasons for doing so are too lengthy to write about here. But, in brief, she was not getting good enough care for her condition and ended up fighting for her life in a hospital. Whew. Scary. And too close for comfort. (Epilogue: she died.) There are similar scary stories about other persons in nursing homes. Because there is no other place to go for long-term care, many, too many, persons with disabilities end up in nursing homes. And it is there they wither away, dying young, dying alone.

In fact, within the disability community, it is often said, "persons with disabilities are warehoused in nursing homes." I am not surprised by that statement any more. The "last stop," as nursing homes are often called, is being recognized worldwide as a poor answer to our final stage in life. Poor, very scary, and outrageously expensive.

I again refer to a "20/20" nursing home horror show that was recently aired. With their hidden cameras, the commonly practiced abuse and neglect were made apparent for all to see. Then, in *Consumer Report's* October 1995 article, "Can Your Loved Ones Avoid a Nursing Home?," a three-part series on caring for the elderly, they discuss some possible alternatives. At best, the report is dismal. And very scary. To quote *Consumer Report's* comment on the provisions found in the offered contracts, "The vagueness of those provisions is tailor-made for abuse and neglect, and it is possible for a facility to manipulate the services to meet its financial objectives rather than the needs of its residents."

Interestingly, the November-December *Mouth*[1] magazine devotes its whole issue to the very unjustness of placing people with disabilities in nursing homes. In fact, *Mouth* magazine laid it out so clearly in this issue, called "You Choose," that it has become a working tool in convincing our politicians that a change is imperative here.

Denmark is one country very aware of the corruption and unnecessary expense of this tragic way to end one's life. Of course, the Danish also are concerned about their own tax loads. The solution? The Danes have placed their elderly citizens and persons with disabilities back into the communities, among a mixed population, among the very young and old, among members of their able and not so able-bodied individuals in society. As a result, in Denmark, there are no ghettos harboring one kind of people. And who pays? The Danish government. It's still far cheaper than Medicare or Medicaid. Talk about common sense.

Writing about my own nursing home experience for the newspapers opened a floodgate of stories from others. One reader wrote, "You [were] one of the lucky ones . . . not until I was subjected to the horror did I believe things could be so bad. I don't think even my husband believed [such was] possible, until I threatened to commit suicide if he didn't get me out of there."

Another reader wrote about her brother being a *"problem"* because he kept bumping the room door with his wheelchair. Obviously, in this institution built in pre-ADA days, the door was a bit narrow to negotiate. And obviously, it is not his fault, nor his problem.

Whenever possible, I like to provide solutions when addressing problems. Fortunately, there are some alternative answers to nursing homes, or what many call the "last stop." From Denver to Denmark, there are some very practical ideas, a couple of them tried and true. And so, I breathe sighs of relief.

In the name of both saving money and maintaining a certain amount of quality, you have the Danish substitute for nursing homes. You have the ADAPT[2] proposal, from an organization headquartered in Denver. Also, you have cohousing groups popping up all over North America, forming a movement toward a new way of living among others.

What all these things have in common is the sharing of responsibility, of being committed to more community involvement, and of caring about the exercise of practical solutions. Translate that last rather important item into saving money. Interestingly, these alternatives to the "last stop" are applicable to every American, persons with disabilities included. Ah, another sigh of relief—another act of inclusion.

I wrote about Denmark dissolving their nursing homes back in the late eighties and returning residents to group homes within their communities. They not only found this cheaper, but they also found it be far more humane. In researching the accessibility of these places, I photographed one. It was a light-filled, clean, non-institutional appearing residence. And a very relaxing ambiance in which to visit as well. Rectangular in shape, this home had a bedroom in every corner. At both ends of the house, situated in between each two bedrooms, was a roomy bathroom, each a minimum twelve feet square. Occupying the center of the home was a kitchen and living/dining room, warmed by an adjoining solarium.

Of course, the house was built on a north-south axis, obtaining maximum solar exposure on its long side for winter heat. Because persons with disabilities and older people tend to move about more slowly, keeping warm in the winter is a challenge. Utilizing solar energy for a home that needs to maximize warmth for its slower-moving residences is a very wise move indeed. And considering that gas and wood heat are both expensive and nonrenewable sources of heat adds to the wisdom of using solar energy.

Because the house is built in a simple rectangle shape and has only one floor, construction costs are kept down. The warmest part of the house is where most of the daily activity happens, in the living/dining room and kitchen, of course. And, as previously mentioned, this home is light-filled with plenty of thermal-paned windows, white walls, and light oak floors. Both the residents and the plants—which are every-where—thrive in this light. This can provide an especially important psychological benefit during their long, dismal winter days. In fact, natural light is considered an immune booster by many professionals in the health field.

Of course, there are no floor-level changes, thereby allowing wheelchairs total freedom of movement. There are no throw rugs for the slow-walker to trip over. All doors are thirty-six inches wide. As a result, no expensive retrofitting is necessary to widen doors nor are there "problem" residents trying to get their too-wide wheelchairs through the too-narrow doors.

Considering that fifty-one percent of Americans are worried about cuts in Medicare, according to a poll reported in the *Albuquerque Journal* on November 3, 1995, saving money is obviously an issue of major concern. This is no surprise. ADAPT has a very practical answer. They say, take twenty-five percent of Medicare's ridiculously wasted dollars and earmark the money for at-home attendant care for persons with disabilities. Because this mostly involves assistance in daily living tasks, such as cooking, eating, dressing, showering, et al., it does not require the use of a professional, nor does it cost as much as a nursing home.

It goes without saying that most of us are happier in our own environments, surrounded by family and friends, surrounded by personal mementos, surrounded by the familiar and not by strangers, nor by odd noises or different routines.

To sum up, the educational organization, Inclusion NM!, leaves us with the question, "What part of *all* don't you understand?" In regard to the "last stop" quandary, it's a good question.

CHAPTER

25

A FEW WORDS ON
BECOMING SAVVY

By now, you probably have a notion that being, or becoming, disabled also means being, or becoming, outspoken, involved. How? We need not look very far. The Ratzkas, the Roberts, the MacGugans are examples.

They are, were, gentle but tireless warriors. They fought, and still fight smart battles, not angry ones. They have demonstrated, and still do demonstrate, disability cool, disability pride. In their lives, the personal has become political; the political, personal.

So how can we do awesome things like ensuring the sensibility and accessibility, into and of, our transit systems? Again, we look at the city of Vancouver, British Columbia, as a shining star—where the voices of advocacy groups were heard early in the planning stages of modernizing their public transportation system. Likewise, one of the most pedestrian-friendly and accessible cities here in the United States is Portland, Oregon. Why? People from all walks were involved in the planning stages, well before from-the-ground-up stuff.

Contacting and maintaining a solid connection with our civic leaders always helps. Educate, educate, and educate. Religiously. Writing letters, endlessly, to our congressmen, the legislators, the president, and others, keeps the awareness up. They should never be let off the hook. They should never forget. We don't. Granted, all of this requires unrelenting work, but nobody else will steer the plow for us. Poet, ecological steward, and activist Gary Snyder was asked in a recent interview if he was tired of talking about politics after over forty years of so doing. He replied,

> Am I tired of talking about it? I'm tired of *doing* it! But hey, you've *got* to keep doing it. That's part of politics, and politics is more than winning or losing at the polls.

So, we, the disability community, need to keep this pressure up, regardless of season, regardless of how tired we are. From our chairs, with our canes, with whatever, we need to learn how to till the earth ourselves. The harder we work, the greater our harvest, no?

The potential is certainly there. According to the Census Bureau, twenty-four percent of voting-age citizens are people with disabilities. Considering that seventy-five percent of all elections are decided by a margin of six to eight percent and that seventy-five percent of these margin votes are done by absentee ballot—a veritable weapon of the disabled voter— we are talking about considerable clout.

There is a shining knight in the ranks of our troops who is not only very aware of this potential, but has also decided to do something about it. His name is Shawn Casey O'Brien and he is the creator of the Unique People's Voting Project (UP).[1] According to a recent (April 1996) *New Mobility* [2] magazine article about O'Brien, UP was created because, as O'Brien says,

> As a nonpartisan, nonprofit voter registration and education project by, for, and of disabled citizens, [we need] to organize disabled citizens so they can protect and promote their civil

rights and economic interests through the ballot box.

O'Brien goes on to explain that we do have a secret weapon: the permanent absentee ballot.

> It gives the voter an easy and convenient way to vote; you get all kinds of election information in advance and it makes it easy to track the disabled vote and its electoral impact. All disabled citizens and their primary caregivers are eligible. So even if you plan to go to the polls, I urge you to use it.

And O'Brien continues,

> If we can get ourselves together electorally, we won't have to fight over things like attendant care. Politicians pay attention to those who vote . . . once we're voting, they'll start paying attention to us.

The underlying message of UP, according to O'Brien, is:

> To tell disabled citizens to have a nobler vision of themselves. Don't think you have to beg legislators to get what you need, or if you ask for too much, you might upset them. We want to upset them — on election day. Our biggest problem is not that the system has beat us down, but we haven't organized ourselves to do the simplest thing — vote in our common interest.

Of course, there will be the droughts, floods, and more. Bravery to continue in the light of the unexpected disaster is forever needed. And, of course, most essential is our humor and likewise our ability to remain soft and pliable. Chogyam Trungpa says that softening and bravery go hand in hand. "Discovering fearlessness comes from working with the softness of the human heart." Otherwise, ". . . bravery is brittle, like a china cup. If you drop it, it will break." So it goes without saying, the combination of courage and tenderness is essential to being a genuine, and tireless, warrior.

But, to be a tireless warrior also means having good tools. It is that basic. To some, a wheelchair is like a pair of shoes, to some a cane is like a third leg, to some a pair of glasses is like a focused camera. To others, a counselor is a breath of fresh air, a hearing aid is a welcomed sound system or a clean environment allows the canary to fly free. But to all, a good fit, the correct length, a compatible match, or a pollution-free environment are most significant. Having the right tool allows us to remain feisty and healthy. Becoming knowledgeable in the use of proper tools is essential to our continued well-being and participation in life.

Good ergonomics, a good fit, is an important feature to anyone's battle for independence and survival. The right fit of things—now that I spend most of my waking hours in the wheelchair or the three-wheel power scooter—is critical for me in order to have continual energy to fight the good battle. I mean, realistically, how far can you continue to hike with a growing blister on your heel from a poorly fitted boot?

In fact, a good fit is recognized as so important in Sweden that they have ergonomic specialists similar to our occupational therapists, who do nothing but fit a device for you. On top of that, Sweden also has centers that provide you with a loaner for a trial period. Free of charge. In testing the product, you can get a feel for whether or not this is an ideal design for you. In other words, you do the choosing. After all, you are the one that uses this tool the most, no? It is also interesting to note that these centers pass on their used, but still very durable, loaners to third world countries, free, when the manufacturers replace these loaners with new, updated versions.

Years ago, when in Sweden, I got a lightweight wheelchair designed by a chair user himself, and tested by many wheelchair users—both big and small, strong and weak—even before it went into production. The chair turns on a dime and is extraordinarily comfortable. It took the ergonomic specialist over two hours to make all the adjustments for me while I was right there, giving her feedback. Getting the right fit requires the crucial personal touch. That is why so many of us refuse to buy shoes through the mail.

With the price of some power wheelchairs approaching that of an automobile, largely paid for by third-party resources here in America, we need to make certain that the final choice is a good one. As when buying a very expensive pair of shoes, you cannot return once worn.

But the horror begins when talking about any piece of durable medical equipment, such as an American-made motorized rickshaw, that was designed without ergonomic considerations. I've used a few. Chances are, and evidence appears, that most were designed and tested by able-bodied males. And a majority of these rickshaws equally are sold by non-users. So right down the line, there are problems due to the lack of experiential awareness. Of course, *if* you have medical insurance, your qualified, knowledgeable occupational/physical therapist or durable medical equipment specialist can help. Meanwhile, back to design, back to carrying on, back to involvement.

In Sweden, there is a company that specializes in the ergonomics of such essential tools, called the Ergonomi Design Gruppen (EDG). Founded in 1979, this cooperatively-owned company is now one of Sweden's largest and oldest consulting firms in the field. Because they are internationally known for their quality ergonomic design of products used by persons with disabilities, I sought them out when in Stockholm. I spent a fascinating afternoon with one of EDG's founders, Maria Benktzon. She emphasized over and over, "Our starting point is the user's knowledge."

For example, their Eat and Drink series are designed to meet the needs of persons with mobility disabilities. Made of high-impact, lightweight plastics and strong, but thin, metal parts, the utensils are easy to use. Too, they are handsome and simple in appearance while being light in weight. Not surprisingly, they have found acceptance among nondisabled users as well. Whether designing or selling, we need to follow EDG's method of never forgetting the true expert—the end user.

The message here is, never underestimate how much you know or can do. Get involved in the fitting of things, participate in any and all possible design projects, speak out, laugh a lot, but be gentle, always, and in all ways. Learn. Become an expert. Exercise savvy knowledge. Then educate, educate, and educate. Religiously. And advocate, but advocate gently. Be pliable. Remember, the soft touch is tolerated far better than the angry slap. Make sure you've got top-notch tools to keep going. And in the words of Winston Churchill, remember, "We must never surrender, never, never, never."

PART FOUR

Life after a Wheelchair

26

THE RISE AFTER
THE STUMBLE

On Losses

We all fall, and that includes professionals like Steve Young of the 49ers, ex-gymnast Nadia Comaneci, and then the ordinary folks, like skiers, joggers, and infants learning to walk. We fall in seriousness and, too, in play. Some falls can be expected and others are very surprising. For a few of us, the fall can be a result of tripping over something not always visible, but there for sure. I often refer to this as a boulder thrown in my small creek of life, backing up its water until the creek can find a new path in which to flow.

To rise after the stumble—it is something we all must do after a stroke, after an auto accident, or after a diagnosis not so pleasant. And truthfully, it is the style of our rising that affects how we will then carry on. But, when the boulder falls, and water backs up, it seems to have stagnated—and in its murkiness, this water seems to lack oxygen, clarity, vitality. It is indeed a crummy feeling, a feeling of being trapped. Darn that boulder. . . . "Why me?" we ask.

"Oh Lord, what is this really about?" we think. I've come to discover these past few years that though the boulder seemed to tumble down the hillside accidentally, nature isn't so accidental. Simple as that. But then, I hate it when some pious person tries to tell me, "There is a reason for this." A reason for the boulder to fall? A reason for cancer? A reason for MS? A reason for rape? A reason for nuclear weapons? A reason for pain, small or great?

Answers, I confess, are no closer, but what is clearer to me now, is the importance of *how* one chooses to rise after such a stumble. Professionals bounce back. They are paid to do so. Skiers relax when they fall. That is part of the sport. They know how to do it well and find it easy enough to get up. Infants try getting up again and again, tears regardless. To walk is an instinct. Granted, we that are unexpectedly flattened are not paid to bounce back, nor do we tend to relax in such a stumble; and alas, instinct does not give much help for a person who is paralyzed to walk again. But there is, somewhere in this low spot, a point where the creek's water can find a path through which to flow again. After all, water always seeks the low point.

I think of Beryl Potter, my host in Toronto the summer of 1989, sans both legs and her right arm, and with a sightless right eye, all due to a freak series of accidents, telling me, "I'm so lucky to be alive." And I think of Dr. Adolf Ratzka of Stockholm, who for five years, beginning at the ripe age of seventeen, was institutionalized after surviving polio. These are only two of the many people who ultimately were willing to dig down and call on their inner resources to rise gracefully after the fall, to allow a low point for the water to flow, and begin once again. As Loren Eiseley said, "If there is magic on this earth, it is contained in water." In their lives and in their magic, the aforementioned people have shown a vibrancy of beautiful resonance—a vibrancy that sparkles like a sun-dappled lake.

I wish I had the know-how and ability to give this vibrancy to all people. But even I struggle on my off days to keep from getting buried too deep. It is a singular struggle, a process that only I can resolve, a solitary job, just as the old axiom puts it, "We are born alone, and too, must die alone." So feel your low point. It is okay. Then discover the flowing vibrancy in your creek—after all, there lies magic in water and in the flow of your life. But just remember one thing: there is no timetable. I share this quote from Rudyard Kipling with you because it has, in many ways, helped me a lot in dealing with my own stumbles:

> If you can meet with triumph and disaster
> And treat those two impostors just the same . . .
> And lose, and start again at your beginning
> And never breathe a word about your loss . . .
> Yours is the earth, and everything that's in it.

On Attitude

In the last decade or so, we have opened our hearts and souls in talking and sharing with others the experience of loss. There are numerous support groups, professionals who are experts in the field, written pieces on this subject, and more. In sources ranging from Kate W. Slagle's excellent book, *Live with Loss*, to Judith Viort's best seller, *Necessary Losses*, plus the superb work and writings by individuals like Stephen Levine and Elisabeth Kübler-Ross, the common denominator of our lives—loss—is shown as something we all experience. We live a loss through separation, divorce, loss of our personhood because of abuse, death of a loved one, loss of our health or our physical abilities, to mention a few. No one is exempt.

None are greater or lesser than the other. They are equal in pain. Yet, we all respond to losses differently. They say as you get older, you can deal with it better. Maybe so and maybe not. Like many, I have endured a number of losses. Some heal within a decent amount of time, and some I deal with on a lifelong basis—or so it seems. I do confess I have not always dealt with them well, but now can respond to them with a greater sense of equanimity. I don't attribute this to the numbers of losses endured. I attribute it more to age.

Age does help to bring about greater understanding and acceptance of the beginning/end cycles in life — that wherever there is a beginning, there is an end. Being that philosophical in understanding does, fortunately, come with age. But this doesn't make a loss any easier. The pain we each endure is still just as great. For those who acquire a disability later on in their lives, dealing with both physical and emotional challenges remains a tall order and demands a long process of recovery, regardless.

Says Susan Rich in a recent *Inside MS* [1] publication about an emotional aspect of her physical disability, "Last week I spoke to a friend . . . we're unable to wear high heels anymore. We talked about what we'd each done with them. She has thrown hers out, and it was a very hard thing to do. I haven't . . . partly because of reluctance to let go of yesterday."

About physical adjustments, writer Andre Dubus, after losing his leg in an accident, says, "When you have always walked, you simply can not imagine all the details of not walking . . ." Overwhelming is about the only word I can think of in describing such a physical loss when combined with advancing age. Friends, family, support groups, and the working professional can help to a certain extent. After the loss, the ensuing grief work can take a longer time under any combined circumstances. And learning to live with these losses is hard, hard work. Unfortunately, it is something we have to do ourselves. No one else can do this for us.

I was recently part of a panel where people with multiple sclerosis talked to those who were newly diagnosed. Excellent advice, good humor, and practical philosophy were meted out. I wish this kind of experiential advice had existed when I was newly diagnosed. One thing everyone stressed is the importance of attitude. In fact, two of us even referred to the same cherished piece on attitude written by Charles Swindle. Swindle says that attitude is more important than the past, education, money, circumstances, or what other people think.

He concludes, "The only thing we can do is play on the one string we have, and that is our attitude."

For a long time, I never realized that attitude is the one string we have. Hindsight now makes that clear. And, unfortunately, for most people, tough conditions tend to worsen when attitude dives. How do we find a positive attitude in ourselves? How do we sustain a good attitude, especially those people with disabilities who, beside handling unrelenting challenges, are encountering the frequently fearful attitudes of others? Or how do we feel, as the French say, "joie de vivre," the joy of living? Where does attitude even come from?

The kind of attitude we have is not inherited. It is simply not in our genes. But parents do play a large role in our young lives cultivating a healthy attitude. Later on in life, the surrounding others can influence our attitude, for better or worse. A good attitude gives us laughter, philosophical insight, and the ability to take ourselves lightly. We become more tolerant of differences. Obstacles become challenges to be met instead of self-defeating deterrents. With a good attitude, we do not tire as easily. And a good attitude helps us to understand our emotional selves more readily.

A good attitude gives one a healthy sense of vitality. Thelma Giomi, an Albuquerque-based clinical psychologist dealing with systemic lupus, says,

> Vitality is being connected with life. Vitality is a
> persistent energy. You will never see as much
> persistent energy as in a well-adjusted person
> with any form of disability. We are connected to
> life. People with chronic health problems
> develop a long patience, a patience of taking the
> first step over and over again as often as it is
> necessary. This is the essence of vitality.

For some, a good attitude is an unspoken gift. For others, a poor attitude is their mode of operation. But we cannot blame our parents for this. When we realize that our own attitude needs a lift, perhaps we can recognize that the responsibility to create a better outlook falls in our own laps. No one else can do this for us. Whether you are an able-bodied soul going through a divorce or a person who is blind, a positive attitude is a lifeline. In fact, a good attitude helps to keep us hale and hearty. This has been known for some time. Even as far back in the seventeenth century, Voltaire said, "I decided I wanted to be happy because it's healthy."

Today, there is Dr. Patch Adams, who believes that the issue of health is not only a better health-care system, but a sillier, happier, and more playful society. With friends and supporters, he founded the Gesundheit Institute[2] years ago. The result? Now the Gesundheit Hospital is being built in West Virginia. Using laughter as a large dose of medicine, Dr. Adams wishes to keep his services light and joyful. Too, for years, the professional health care staff at the Institute have been providing health care services free. The number one prescription? Humor, joy, and laughter. Sound unreal? Then read *Gesundheit!* (P. Adams, Healing Arts Press, 1993), a must for anyone in, or interested in, the healing arts, including all staff and students at any university hospital.

Attitude encompasses so much of our lives, in so many ways, among so many walks. A friar at the Graymoor Monastery in Garrison, New York, wrote the following:

> If I had my life to live over, I'd try to make more
> mistakes next time. I would relax. I would
> limber up. I would be sillier than I have been on
> this trip. I know of a very few things I would
> take seriously. I would be crazier. I would be less
> hygienic. I would take more chances. I would
> take more trips. I would climb more mountains,
> swim more rivers and watch more sunsets. I
> would eat more ice cream and less beans. I
> would have actual troubles and fewer imaginary
> ones. . . . Oh, I have had my moments and, if I
> had it to do over again, I'd have more of them.
> In fact, I'd try to have nothing else. Just mo-
> ments, one after another, instead of living so
> many years ahead each day. . . . If I had it to do
> over again, I would go places and do things and

travel lighter than I have. If I had my life to live over, I would start barefooted earlier in the spring and stay that way later in the fall. I would play hooky more. I wouldn't make such good grades except by accident. I would ride on more merry-go-rounds. I'd pick more daisies.

About laughs, Dr. Carol Gill, a psychologist and disability rights activist, says that crip humor is a vital component to our accepting ourselves and creating a healthy attitude about our situations. She says,

> . . . the next time you share a joke with a disabled friend or laugh at a disability cartoon or comedy routine, take the time to consider the function and value of disability humor. It serves to articulate our experience, express beliefs and feelings, affirm our worth, define who we are, assert our durability and power, and draw us together. In sum, it helps us live.

On the Quality of Life

Is there life after a wheelchair? Now, I can say, "Absolutely." But, right after I started to use the chair, I bought into the notion, "Better dead than disabled." Fortunately, my suicide attempt failed. But the recovery was long and slow and painful. And in many ways, it was one big diversion from continuing to grow, to live, to learn.

They say you always learn by hindsight. But if your suicide attempt works, there will be no hindsight to be had. So can I beg one thing of you? Before drawing conclusions, let hindsight play a part of any decision. There is no reason to buy into society's aphorisms. You are you, not society. Experience tells me that the motto, "It's better to be dead than disabled," does not belong to the disability community's philosophy. More than likely, the motto was coined by some able-bodied wimp, a gutless, fearful wimp, to be more precise. I wish such understanding had been part of my foresight instead of hindsight.

Learn from high-level quadriplegics who need a ventilator for help in breathing. The April 1996 issue of *New Mobility (NM)* magazine,[3] reports that such persons feel their quality of life is fine, while health professionals and others (read that as able-bodied people, who do not need ventilators) consistently underestimate the level of life satisfaction among such individuals. *NM* got this information from a forthcoming book, *Independent Living and Quality of Life among Persons Who Use Ventilators,* written by Margaret A. Nosek, Ph.D. and S. Ann Holmes, M.D. *NM* says, "Both authors are ventilator users themselves." So who is to judge about life satisfaction? Right. Those living their own lives, not others, not society. Keep this in mind as part of your foresight and let it be lovely hindsight as well.

ON EXERCISING YOUR
SPIRITUAL MUSCLE

I once gave a talk: "Exercising Your Spiritual Muscle—You Lose What You Don't Use." Then, shortly following the talk, I received an issue of *New Mobility*[1] magazine *(NM)* in the mail. Their theme in that issue? "Becoming Whole: Healing from the Inside Out." Nothing like being trendy. Better yet: nothing like being aware—of yourself, of the positiveness of disability, of your own spiritual muscle. *NM* introduces their series of articles on becoming whole by saying:

> While all lives are journeys, life with a disability can be a particularly jarring one. Because a lot is taken away, we have a lot to recover. Because we aren't cured, we have to heal. Because parts of us no longer work, we need to identify the parts that still do. Because disability comes with so much that we don't want, we have to rediscover what it is we do want. We have to become whole.

In introducing the first article, by researcher and writer Carolyn Vash, *NM* posits, "Maybe disability—dare we say it?—has some spiritual utility." Though risking a pat rational answer as to the whys of our becoming disabled, the idea is certainly worth thinking about.

In the talk on exercising your spiritual muscle, I began by saying:

> In the last couple of years, my body has gotten weaker. It has been more of a physical task. I've fallen and I've done things that have required stitches, that have required minor surgery, that have required plain old physical recovery, and that have required more adjusting—always more adjusting.

People would come up all the time and say, "Karen, I don't know how you do it." To that I would always answer, "If you're there, you do it." And lately, I realize I've been saying, "Oh, yeah. I've been getting weaker physically, but my spirit is fine." And that got me thinking, "Why is my spirit fine?" Part of the reason why it's fine is that I've learned to take myself lightly. I've learned to laugh a lot. It helps to view the vagaries of life with a humorous slant.

And laughter certainly helps to alleviate any pain. In this vein, I never forget the axiom, "She who laughs, lasts." Dr. Carol Gill, a psychologist and disability rights activist, talks about the healing value of humor. Dr. Gill reinforces my view that laughter is a phenomenal stress-reliever, especially within disability circles. It is also empowering, acknowledging that you are part of all this and can speak the language while winking one eye.

In her *NM* article, "From Transcendence To Transformation," Carolyn Vash says,

> Common to all cultures is the recognition that a massive interruption of life patterns is a prime requisite to spiritual evolution.

And in my talk I said,

> I am disabled. So what? I cannot spend time
> trying to figure out what I did wrong in my past
> life that led to this so-called present day karma.
> I'm not going to worry about that. There's too
> much going on. There's a lot of life in front of me.

Carolyn Vash later refers to Rev. Terry Cole-Whittaker's 1982 book, *What You Think of Me Is None of My Business,* by stating, "She [Cole-Whittaker] suggests the possibility of transcending the evaluations other people make of you." I could not agree more. It's a good thing to do. At one point in my talk, I remarked, "You know, it's like, I've got this label and I always thought the label of 'handicapped' was a label I had to accept. What a bunch of nonsense."

I can't walk. So what? It's okay. Our minds are so busy and full of criticizing ourselves, criticizing others. There is that wonderful Japanese saying, "If you criticize someone out there, look at yourself first." So I do. In his *NM* article, "Supermarket Spirituality: Making Sense of the Illogical and Unexplainable," writer and counselor Richard Holicy says,

> Maybe it wasn't my problem, but theirs. . . .
> After a couple of years of this, it finally dawned
> on me that perhaps the way to transcendence,
> true transcendence, was to transcend all these
> buttheads and get on with my life.

I concluded my talk by saying,

> So, that's a little bit on exercising your spiritual
> muscle. You get your body, you get yourself, you
> get your mind out of the way. The only part that
> I recommend you don't leave out of the way is
> your heart. Follow your heart. Listen to your
> heart. Let your heart express itself. And don't
> worry about what others think.

NM interviewed the late Ken Keyes, a major figure in the personal growth field for years, who died recently at the age of seventy-five. He had been quadriplegic since 1946, after a bout with polio. At one point in the interview, he explains his transcendence,

> And as that understanding [being able to do the
> things he is able to do] gradually worked into
> my mind, and got stronger and stronger, I saw
> that being disabled is just one more thing and
> not really a big thing. Just one more thing.

NM concluded the series with an article by Richard Louis Bruno, "Disabled Man: Oxymoron or Ubermensch?" In this article, Bruno writes about Robert Bly's referring to the myth that physical disability gives its owner a compassionate heart. Says Bruno, "Mythic figures, including Jacob, Oedipus, and even Jesus, were said to walk with a limp . . . [and] in a flash of insight, I reached the inescapable conclusion: God is a high-level quad." I like that.

Around this same time, I had a dream. It was lousy. But revealing. Everyone in the dream had AIDS. Some had already died. Some were in the final throes of the disease. Some were barely showing symptoms. But all of us knew we had it and were going to die from it. We were in a natural setting, almost like a camp. It felt much like Asilomar. For those of you unfamiliar with this place, a retreat center in California, imagine a forested cove with sandy grounds by the ocean front along the northern coast.

There were lots of ice plants growing on the grounds. Known to grow profusely in such settings, these succulents had colorful flowers that would close at night and spread wide open in the warmth of the day. The cabins where most of us slept—some camped outdoors—were nestled back in the protective environs of the nearby forest groves. Interestingly, despite the natural ruggedness, the place was accessible, laced by hard-packed paths that even remained so in rainy weather. Don't ask me how. It was a dream.

I go into great length describing this setting because of its revelatory nature. Growing up, I attended Quaker retreats at Asilomar. And when dealing with something as difficult as AIDS was in the dream, as disabling as this condition actually is, and as final as death equally is, the need to exercise our spiritual strength is quite obvious. So Asilomar naturally was a perfect symbol.

That they say, "We age into disability," also makes sense. In the dream we were all looking at the inevitability of our death, and we should equally look into the probable possibility of our becoming disabled, in one form or another, sooner or later.

And as in the dream we had an innate understanding of just how inevitable our demise was, is, there should be a parallel understanding that disability, or becoming disabled, is equally part of the norm. With such thinking, architects would be designing buildings differently. If they say, "Buildings shape our lives," we can now assert our lives will shape buildings.

With such understanding, laws like the Americans with Disabilities Act would not be necessary. As in the dream, in the commonality of our all having AIDS—despite our different ages and backgrounds—we automatically understood the needs of one another. Laws mandating the addressing of such needs, of course, would not be necessary. In reality, such legal riprap would be a waste of time. As in the dream, we instead would deal with the spiritual. Our need to be strong in the face of the unknown is more crucial than many think.

In the dream, my family and friends were comforting and supporting one another. There was a display of photos of those who have just passed away. It was a nonverbal announcement and reminder, a reminder of that person and what is still to come for us.

So in real life, "when this you see, remember me". . . as I struggle to open the too-heavy door. Why not automatic door openers? Does not the pregnant mother, the business person loaded with binders of paperwork, or the student carrying stacks of books equally benefit by automatic door openers? How many times have you taken your full shopping cart out to the car and have been grateful for, or even have noticed, the automatic door openers?

Remember me as I am absent because the entry steps will not accommodate my round shoes, the wheelchair. Or remember me without my friend because the hall has just been sprayed with pesticide to get rid of unwanted critters, the poison making her rather ill in short order.

Remember me as I do not attend the opera because my friend, an opera freak, cannot drive since he is blind, and there is no accessible public transportation we can take together.

Remember me for refusing to go to a public forum because there are no sign language interpreters, discriminating against members of the deaf community from participating. I no longer tolerate such injustice.

Remember me as I concentrate to appreciate what the child trying to tell me despite his communicative disorder. Remember me as I read up and study more about mental illnesses so I can be both more understanding and compassionate.

Remember me when you laugh, cry or get dissed, because I am as human as you are and have much the same feelings. Then you'll find me opening wide like flowers do in midday's warmth.

Remember me when I have a dream . . . we all do.

APPENDICES

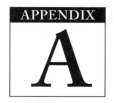

A

HOW TO MAKE A PUBLIC EVENT ACCESSIBLE

There are many public events occurring every day. And there are many of us living with a disability, who would like to attend an event but cannot do so because of inaccessibility. Ironically, event organizers are constantly pondering how to increase their attendance while often ignoring accessibility issues. Yet, current figures estimate twenty percent of Americans to have some kind of disability. Ignore accessibility needs, and you automatically eliminate a certain constituency from attending. While I believe the above percentage is low for a variety of reasons, it is time that event organizers recognize this as an untapped market waiting to be acknowledged. A gold mine if you ask me.

There is absolutely no reason to believe that the disability community is neither interested nor unwilling nor lacking in the discretionary income to participate. Granted, some members of the disability community may not have as much money to dole out because some are without jobs—but this is not true of all. And what about those who are retired and simply have been slowed down by age? Or money notwithstanding, what about the enthusiastic support such individuals can offer?

Do we not vote, pay taxes, attend PTA meetings, laugh, cry, go to movies, and shop like anyone else? Do persons with disabilities not have children, dreams, or aspirations like all of us? How would you feel about Grandma not attending your child's musical concert because it involved going up steps?

Or is the ADA (Americans with Disabilities Act) frustrating you too much, so you choose to risk ignoring it instead? How about simply utilizing common sense to ensure a modicum of accessibility to maximize attendance? In doing so, everyone would win. There are a few obvious things to do. As follows, check:

- Is handicap parking available and are there ramps up the sidewalks leading to the main entrance?

- Make sure there are no steps, anywhere one needs to go the duration of the event.

- Make sure doors are wide enough, preferably with a minimum of thirty-two inches actual clearance.

- Are doors easy to open? If not, can't you assign a "Greeter" to open the door while saying, "Welcome"? After all, the bigger hotels do so and with good reason, whether the guests have luggage or no luggage in tow.

- Is there an accessible pathway, at least thirty-two inches wide, all the way to the meeting room, the rest room, and the drinking fountain?

- Is the bathroom accessible with at least one toilet stall big enough and with the essential grab bars? Don't laugh. We can all use such an accommodation, anytime, anywhere. After all, we are all human.

The grab bars are an issue of safety. It's no fun falling with your pants down because of the lack of support. Don't laugh again. It once happened to yours truly. Five stitches later, I can say I got off easy.

- Check the doors to the rest rooms. The same guidelines apply as above. Nothing like having to relieve yourself, but not be able open the door . . .

- For the deaf, is there a sign language interpreter or two (one to spell the other—it's incredibly hard work)?

- Also, provide additional material in print to take home and later read to make sure nothing has been missed.

- For the blind community or those with low vision, is there an alternative program in Braille, large print, or, if lengthy, on tape?

- And are service dogs allowed in?

Remember the bumper sticker, "Make it happen!"? Do it. After all, it's the law.

Now, I'd like to address some not-so-obvious concerns. But because these concerns are not so evident does not mean, in any way, they are less important. A well-prepared public event for all attendees is a success in itself. Dealing with subtle concerns creates an equalizing platform which encourages full participation. Some of these additional, and not-so-obvious, concerns involve lighting, sound, and allergies. Yes, allergies.

As mentioned before, the National Academy of Sciences in Air Pollutants estimated far back as 1981 that up to fifteen percent of the United States population suffer from chemical sensitivities. Many years later, I believe this figure is much higher. Yet, despite all, here in the United States, we seldom recognize or even acknowledge the impact, and widespread prevalence, of environmental illnesses or multiple chemical sensitivities (EI/MCS) among members of our society. It is about time we do. People with EI/MCS react in varying degrees to many man-made agents such as solvents, fragrances, drugs, cosmetics, auto/industrial emissions, pesticides, herbicides, anycide for that matter. Many individuals with EI/MCS encounter a host of challenges not only in getting to an event. Often they are stopped short of participating at the public event itself because of the numerous barriers encountered there.

Starting at the ground floor, a newly installed rug reeking of the formaldehyde used in the glue to install it can be a most annoying, and even deadly, barrier. Have you ever thought about the crackerjack headache you get after spending some time in a space with a newly installed rug? It's a very mild response, believe me. New carpeting not only affects those with EI/MCS, but often triggers a reaction in those who previously have experienced no allergic response before. Formaldehyde does that, anytime, almost any place.

Here where I live, the city hall is sprayed periodically with an insecticide to keep it free of unwanted critters. Don't breathe. This is a common practice everywhere across the country, city halls often being in older buildings. Make the staff aware of this problem, and try to work out a compromise. If nothing else, request that any work be done after the event, but well before the next public event. If this cannot be resolved, notices should be posted outside the entrance acknowledging that the spraying has occurred on such and such a date.

Designate an area in which people can sit free from others who have slathered on their favorite after-shave lotion or perfume, or have sprayed their coif. After all, people with EI/MCS can be anyone, your mom, dad, partner, friend.

Make sure the lighting is good. I have excellent vision, but simply refuse trying to read anything in dim lighting. Too, there are those with low vision who need the bright lights to see where they are going. Unnecessary accidents often occur in poorly lit areas. More often than you think.

Sitting in the back row, can you easily hear the speaker? And is the actual event locale quiet? Or do you need to close the door(s) to shut out background noise? For those of us who wear hearing aids, background noise can be most deafening.

Advertise that this public event is accessible. Leave a phone number (including a TTY number for the deaf or hard of hearing) one can call to inquire about details or any other special need that might be necessary.

Meanwhile, do make your public event accessible. Remember, it's the law.

B

HOW TO EFFECTIVELY DEAL WITH INJUSTICE

To level out the mountains of injustice that so complicate the lives of individuals with disabilities, a few words of advice. Let me start out by reminding you of the oft-said axiom, "God gave us burdens—and shoulders." Much as we may feel overwhelmed by the burdens of injustice, the load is ours to carry, no matter how we cut it.

Top-notch lawyers or ADA (Americans with Disabilities Act) consultants may be great, but they are not always a panacea to our burdens. Why? First of all, money. How many of us can afford their services? Second, they too are overwhelmed. Third, working with others usually means working things into their schedules, not ours.

So, more often than not, we remain saddled with the burdens, let alone just trying to get through the day. Remember, it was Mother Teresa who said, "I know God gave me burdens. I just wish He wouldn't trust me so much." Laughter, tears, and weariness set aside, to resolve any injustice, the work is really up to us. But, the good news is that we are not alone.

I speak from personal experience as I have been through a few personal battles, daily survival, fatigue, and more notwithstanding. How did I do my homework?

To begin, we must become gophers. We must dig down, deep, turning over every stone in the process, to find our facts. We begin doing this by temporarily making the phone book our bible. Have you ever looked at the information guide in first part of your yellow pages? However, do keep in mind that there are a couple of drawbacks to any phone book listing. One is that you do not find much in the way of alternative help. For that you need to go to your local health food stores and begin searching there. The other drawback is that items are not always listed under the category you might think most likely. To wit, in one big city's phone book, "Senior Well-Being" includes listings such as "Attitudes toward Sex," "Self-Esteem/Wellness," "Grief," "Depression," and "Drug and Alcohol Dependency." All these categories could equally fall under "Disability Concerns," a nonexisting category in most guides.

Regardless, poor categories, recorded message or not, remember one thing always leads to the next. So don't give up—ever. And when actually talking to a person, there are a couple of things to keep in mind.

First, talk early in the morning, when you are freshest and most full of patience. Keep your calls brief, to the point, and pleasant. I cannot underscore enough the importance of being courteous. You never know. You may have to call this person back. And write down the names of those in which you speak. Everyone. Without fail. Also, try to get their job title or the department in which they work. Again, you never know.

Remember, be brief. Do not saddle the other person on the phone with your plight. If you are angry, frustrated, or full of grief, forget calling. Instead, write. Get it all out, don't mail this to anyone, and then, take a nap. That naps are required is my motto. Start again the next day when refreshed.

Because all calling is to be accomplished in the morning, your research, such as perusing the phone book or reading any literature gathered from your local health food store, can be done in the afternoon or early evening when you are resting.

Keep your notes—religiously. Correspondence? Keep a copy of both incoming and outgoing letters—religiously. You never know. Because you may have to pull up one of these items, which invariably you will find yourself doing, do a good job of filing all, from day one.

And last, but not least, no matter with whom you are speaking, ask, "Are there any other resources I should be checking out?" You never know.

As mentioned, perseverance and patience are tools necessary to accomplish any modicum of successful research in our digging for justice. So what are our resources?

Before listing a few national resources, I'd like to quote a piece of advice from the *Pocket Guide to Federal Help for Individuals with Disabilities* (U.S. Department of Education, Office of Special Education and Rehabilitation Services, Rm. 3132, Switzer Bldg., Wash., DC 20202). It says,

> Remember, not every service is available and not every person can be helped 100 percent. Keep in mind that every year new programs begin and old ones end, particularly at the state and local levels. Keep in touch with your contacts and stay as aware as you can, through reading and talking to knowledgeable people about what is happening in the area of services to individuals with disabilities.

Add to that: keep in touch with each other. Share. You know the old rhetoric: "There is power in numbers." What works for you may very well work for others. So share. Share. Share.

On the national level, the Americans with Disabilities Act (ADA) of 1990 guarantees equal rights for people with disabilities in employment, public services, public accommodations, and telecommunications.

For more specific information, contact the sources listed in the following table.

Information on	Source
ADA requirements affecting employment	Equal Employment Opportunity Commission 1801 L St., N.W. Washington, DC 20507 (202) 663-4900 (800) 800-3302 (TDD)
Transportation	Department of Transportation 400 Seventh St., S.W. Washington, DC 20590 (202) 366-9305 (202) 755-7687 (TDD)
Accessible design in new construction and alterations	Architectural and Transportation Barriers Compliance Board 1331 F St., N.W., Ste. 1000 Washington, DC 20004 800-USA-ABLE 800-993-2223 (TDD)
Telecommunications	Federal Communications Commission 1919 M St., N.W. Washington, DC 20554 (202) 632-7260 (202) 632-6999 (TDD)
Public Services and Public Accommodations	Office on the Americans with Disabilities Act Civil Rights Division U.S. Department of Justice P.O. Box 66118 Washington, DC 20035 (202) 514-0301 (202) 514-0383 (TDD)

On the local level, it can be hoped, you have obtained some numbers from the above listings. Try any independent living resource center. Better yet, visit these places. Often, you will find good resources on their bulletin boards. Contact your specific support group or agency. Call your local protection and advocacy organization. Call United Way. Ask. Ask. Ask. There is never an end to finding out about things.

And remember, as Martin Luther King said, "Injustice anywhere is a threat to justice everywhere."

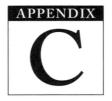

C

QUESTIONS FOR DISCUSSING SEX AND DISABILITIES

- Would you like to be treated differently if you were disabled in an accident?

- Why do you think people feel uneasy when they discuss or hear the term "sexuality?"

- How can we achieve greater frankness and realism in our discussions of sexuality and intimate relations?

- What is sexuality for you (feelings, sex drive, man, woman, reproduction, nearness, desire)? Choose among these and other concepts.

- What do you think about masturbation? Provides sexual excitement/release by own stimulation of the genitals? Petting in different kinds of relationships?

- Are your attitudes positive, negative or neutral?

- Have opinions (yours and society's) changed since you were a teenager? If so, why?

- When did you discover that boys and girls are treated differently? What did your parents say? How did you talk about sex at home? How did you talk about sex in school? What were you ignorant about?

- What do you think most people think? The man should be the most active partner? The woman should be the most active partner?

- How is it in practice?

- Would the answers be different if one partner had a disability?

- A person with a disability may constantly require help in different ways. Does the need for help influence your attitude towards his/her sexuality?

- What do you think about pornography for persons with disabilities who have difficulties in achieving sexual satisfaction and need extra stimulation?

- Where does integrity come in?

- When do you even begin to talk about sex?

- How do you regard sexuality among disabled and non-disabled adolescents? Is there any difference?

- How do you think the subject of relationships and sexuality be approached between
  - doctors and patient?
  - the patient and staff member which she/he has the best contact?
  - parent and child?

or do you just let sleeping dogs lie? Any other opinions?

- How are the questions handled in your private life, at work, in other settings?

- What support can we give to parents of children and adolescents with disabilities?

- What support can we give to a newly disabled person who wonders whether he or she will always have to live alone?

- When someone in your family becomes disabled, this can lead to changes in different areas. For example:

  - the relationship between spouses and partners

  - the division of responsibilities in the home

  - the children

  - relationships between family and friends

  - finances, working life

  - opportunities for getting out, etc.

- Which of these changes do you think is most urgent to talk about? Select them.

Chapter 1. On Disability and Language

1. *The Standard Rules*, 1994, Disabled Persons Unit, Department for Policy Coordination and Sustainable Development, United Nations, Room DC2-1302, New York, NY 10017.

2. *The Ragged Edge*, P.O. Box 145, Louisville, KY 40201. This publication was formerly called *The Disability Rag & Resource*.

Chapter 2. Seeing the Barriers

1. Concrete Change, 1371 Metropolitan Ave., SE, Atlanta, GA 30316.

2. Yoshida, Clara Ako, *Three Stage Housing for Old People, Report of the 2nd International Expert Seminar on Building Non-Handicapping Environments: Renewal of Inner Cities*, The Royal Institute of Technology, 1987.

3. *Computer Resources for People with Disabilities*, The Alliance for Technology Access, Hunter House, 1994.

Chapter 8. Women and Disabilities

1. Berkeley Planning Associates, 440 Grand Ave., Suite 401, Oakland, CA 94610. This organization was formerly called the Pacific Research and Training Alliance.

2. Society for Disability Studies, Suffolk University, Sawyer School of Management, Dept. of Public Management, Eight Ashburton Place, Boston, MA 02108-2770.

3. World Institute on Disability, 510 Sixteenth St., Suite 100, Oakland, CA 94612.

4. DisAbled Women's Network (DAWN), 160 The Esplanade, Apt. 161, Toronto, Ontario, M5A 3T2, Canada.

Chapter 10. Education

1. Centre for Integrated Education & Community, 24 Thorne Cres., Toronto, Ontario, M6H 2S5, Canada.

2. California State University, School of Education, Division of Special Education, 5151 State University Drive, Los Angeles, CA 90032.

Chapter 11. Accessible Housing

1. Planke, Julie. "A Barrier-Free Environment," *Canadian Workshop*, Vol. 12, No. 6, March, 1989, p.54.

2. Ratzka, Adolf. *The Costs of Disabling Environments*, Swedish Council for Building Research, 1984.

3. Laurie, Gini. "European Concepts of Independent Living," *Rehabilitation World*, Spring-Summer 1981, p.44.

4. Weiss-Lindencrona, Hanne. *From "Barrierfication" Towards the "Barrier-Freecation" of Inner Cities*, a report done for The Royal Institute of Technology, 1987, p. 131.

5. Yoshida, Clara Ako, *Three Stage Housing for Old People, Report of the 2nd International Expert Seminar on Building Non-Handicapping Environments: Renewal of Inner Cities*, The Royal Institute of Technology, 1987.

6. The Cohousing Network, P.O. Box 2584, Berkeley, CA 94702.

Chapter 13. Recreation and Leisure

1. Leisurability Publications, Inc., 36 Bessemer Court, Unit 3, Concord, Ontario L4K 3C9, Canada.

2. American Horticultural Therapy Association, 3628 Christopher Ave., Gathesburg, MD 20879.

3. Seeds of Change, P.O. Box 15700, Santa Fe, NM 87506.

Chapter 14. On Travel, Vacations, Naps, and Then Some

1. Travelin' Talk, P.O. Box 3534, Clarksville, TN 37043.

2. Mobility International USA, P.O. Box 3551-C, Eugene, OR 97403.

3. Guide published by Mobility International USA.

4. *New Mobility*, P.O. Box 15518, North Hollywood, CA 91615.

Chapter 16. Aging

1. *New Mobility*, P.O. Box 15518, North Hollywood, CA 91615.

2. National Spinal Cord Injury Association, 545 Concord Ave., Suite 29, Cambridge, MA 02138.

Chapter 17. Diet, Exercise, and Health

1. Jimmie Huega Center, P.O. Box 5919, Avon, CO 81620.

Chapter 19. Sex

1. *New Mobility*, P.O. Box 15518, North Hollywood, CA 91615.

2. *It's Okay!*, Sureen Publications and Productions, P.O. Box 23102, 124 Welland Ave., St. Catharines, Ontario L2R 7P6, Canada.

3. Charcot-Marie-Tooth International, One Springbank Drive, St. Catharines, Ontario L2S 2K1, Canada.

4. Nordqvist, Inger. *Sexuality and Disability: A Matter that Concerns All of Us.* 1986. The Swedish Institute for the Handicapped, Box 303, S-161 26 Bromma, Sweden.

Chapter 24. The Last Stop

1. *Mouth*, 61 Brighton St., Rochester, NY 14607.

2. National ADAPT, P.O. Box 9598, Denver, CO 80203.

Chapter 25. A Few Words on Becoming Savvy

1. The Unique People's Voting Project, 40 Brooks Ave. #2, Venice, CA 90291. Phone: 310-392-3176, or e-mail upvote@aol.com.

2. *New Mobility*, P.O. Box 15518, North Hollywood, CA 91615.

Chapter 26. The Rise after the Stumble

1. *Inside MS*, National Multiple Sclerosis Society, 733 3rd Ave., New York, NY 10017.

2. Gesundheit Institute, 1630 Robert Walker Place, Arlington, VA 22207.

3. *New Mobility*, P.O. Box 15518, North Hollywood, CA 91615.

Chapter 27. On Exercising Your Spiritual Muscle

1. *New Mobility*, P.O. Box 15518, North Hollywood, CA 91615.

Volcano Press Titles

Learning to Live without Violence: *A Handbook for Men* $15.95
by Daniel Jay Sonkin, Ph.D. and Michael Durphy, M.D.

Aprendir a Vivir Sin Violencia. Spanish edition of *Learning* $14.95
to Live Without Violence

Learning to Live without Violence: *Worktape* (2 C-60 cassettes) $15.95
by Daniel Jay Sonkin, Ph.D. and Michael Durphy, M.D.

The Counselor's Guide to Learning to Live without Violence $29.95
by Daniel Jay Sonkin, Ph.D., hardcover

Family Violence and Religion: *An Interfaith Resource Guide* $29.95
Compiled by the staff of Volcano Press, hardcover

The Physician's Guide to Domestic Violence: *How to ask* $10.95
the right questions and recognize abuse (another way to save a life)
by Ellen Taliaferro, M.D. and Patricia R. Salber, M.D.

Walking on Eggshells: *Practical Counsel for Women In or* $8.95
Leaving a Violent Relationship by Dr. Brian Ogawa

Every Eighteen Seconds: *A Journey Through Domestic Violence* $8.95
by Nancy Kilgore

Sourcebook for Working with Battered Women $17.95
by Nancy Kilgore

Battered Wives by Del Martin $12.95

Conspiracy of Silence: *The Trauma of Incest* by Sandra Butler $13.95

Menopause, Naturally: *Preparing for the Second Half of Life,* $14.95
Updated, by Sadja Greenwood, M.D., M.P.H.

Period by JoAnn Gardner-Loulan, Bonnie Lopez and $9.95
Marcia Quackenbush

Wars I Have Seen by Esther Silverstein Blanc $12.95

Goddesses by Mayumi Oda $14.95